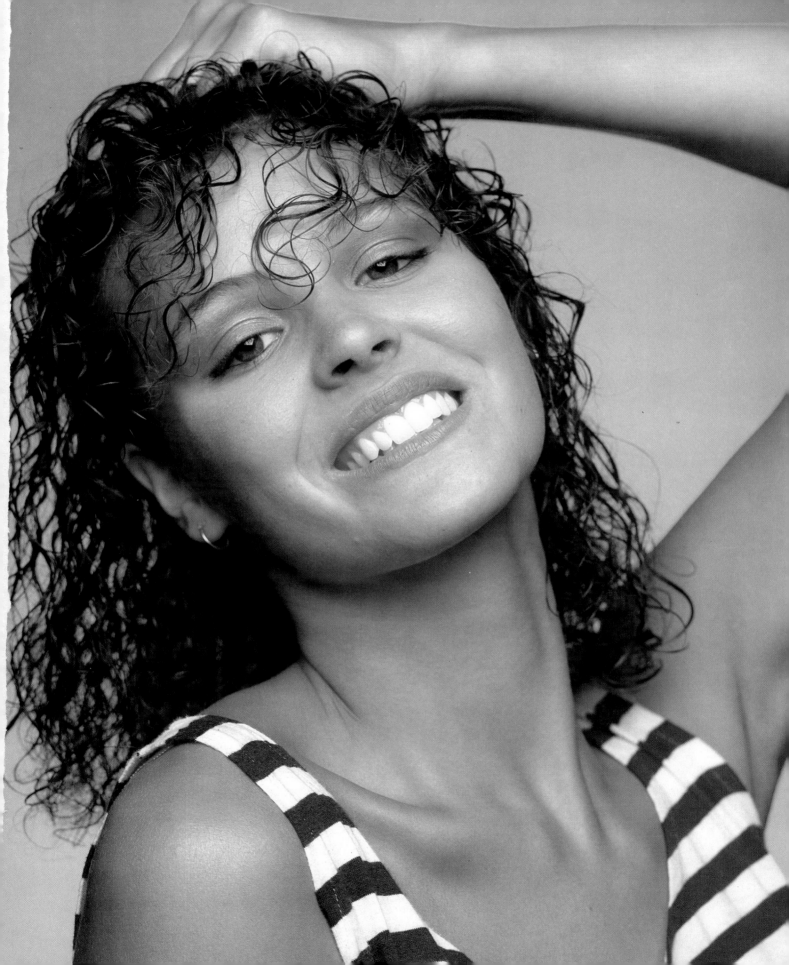

This edition published in 1992 by
Tiger Books International PLC, London
© 1985 Coombe Books
Printed and bound in Hong Kong
1 85501 198 0

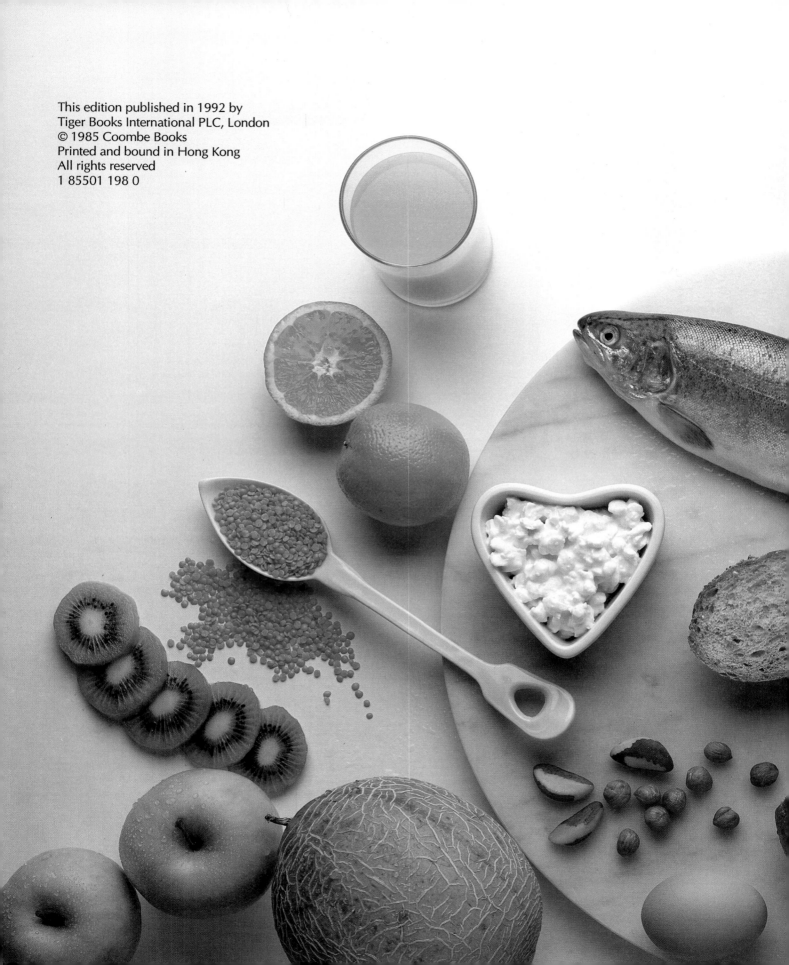

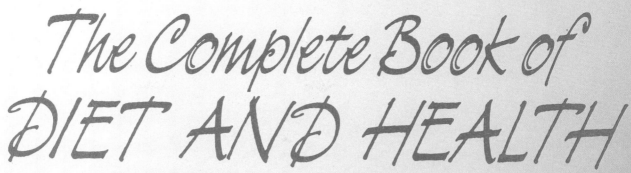

The Complete Book of
DIET AND HEALTH

Miriam Polunin

TIGER BOOKS INTERNATIONAL
LONDON

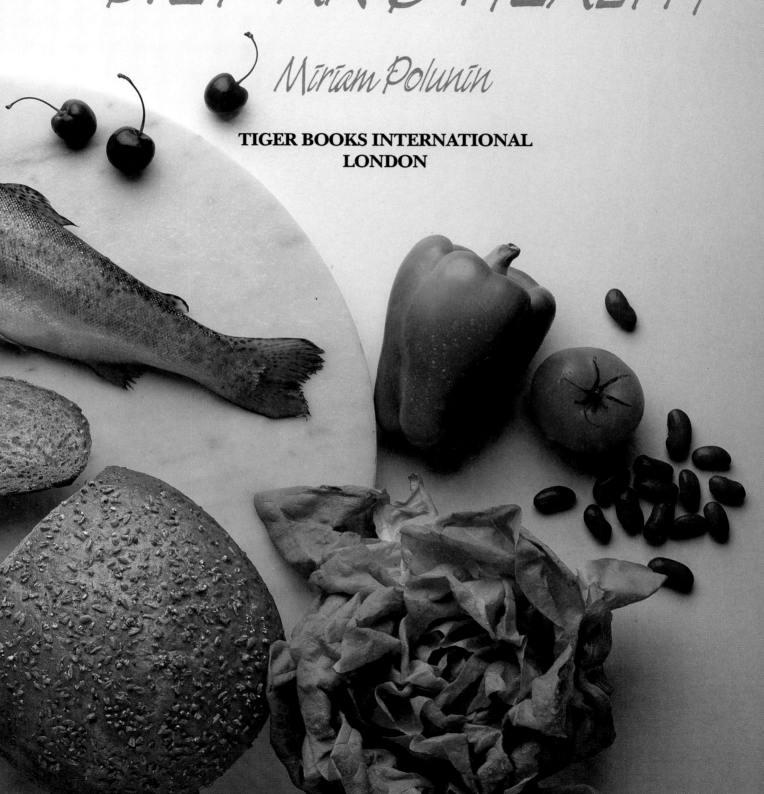

4

Contents

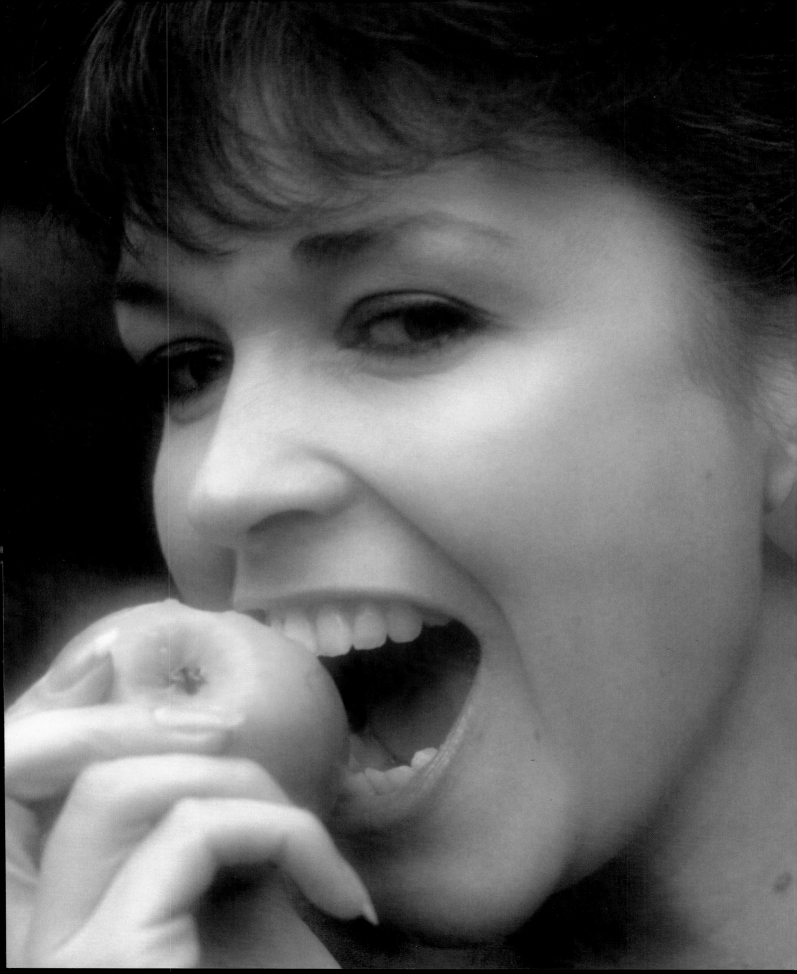

Introduction

Good health is one of the most precious possessions you can have, but if you think it's just a matter of luck, think again.

It's true that you inherit from your parents characteristics which will influence your health, but many illnesses – or plain lack of 'bounce' – have nothing to do with luck. They are the direct result of our own style of living. That means the food we eat, the amount and type of exercise we take, and our attitudes towards life. They all work together and they are all our choice. That's encouraging, because it means we can change them, once we become aware of how they affect our health. Whatever your health when born, you can make the most of it. Good health really does make a difference, and the health you build for yourself can help give your children a better start in life.

This book is about how to choose a life style – particularly a style of eating – that will do most to improve and maintain your health. In the process you'll also be helping your looks, and before you give up any idea of dazzling the world, take a look at some famous good-lookers. You'll find that their features are often no better than those of people around you. What often makes the difference is an inner sparkle that makes them appear outstandingly attractive, even if they have far smaller eyes, bigger ears, or a weaker chin than the accepted ideal.

Inner sparkle is partly tied to personality,

Far right and right: life isn't fair in what looks and physique we inherit. But your own attitude to life – positive or negative – and the health habits you choose, are just as important to your health and appearance.

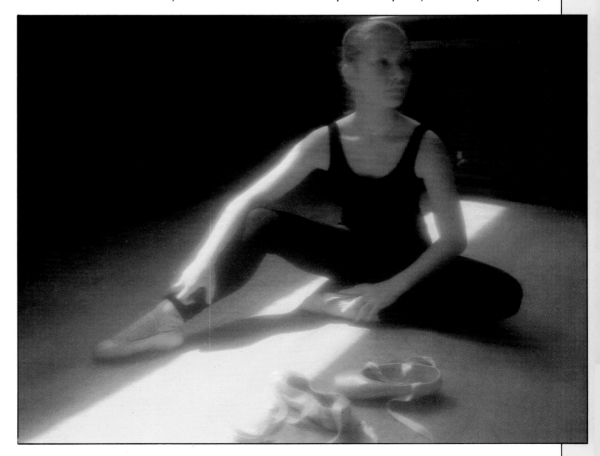

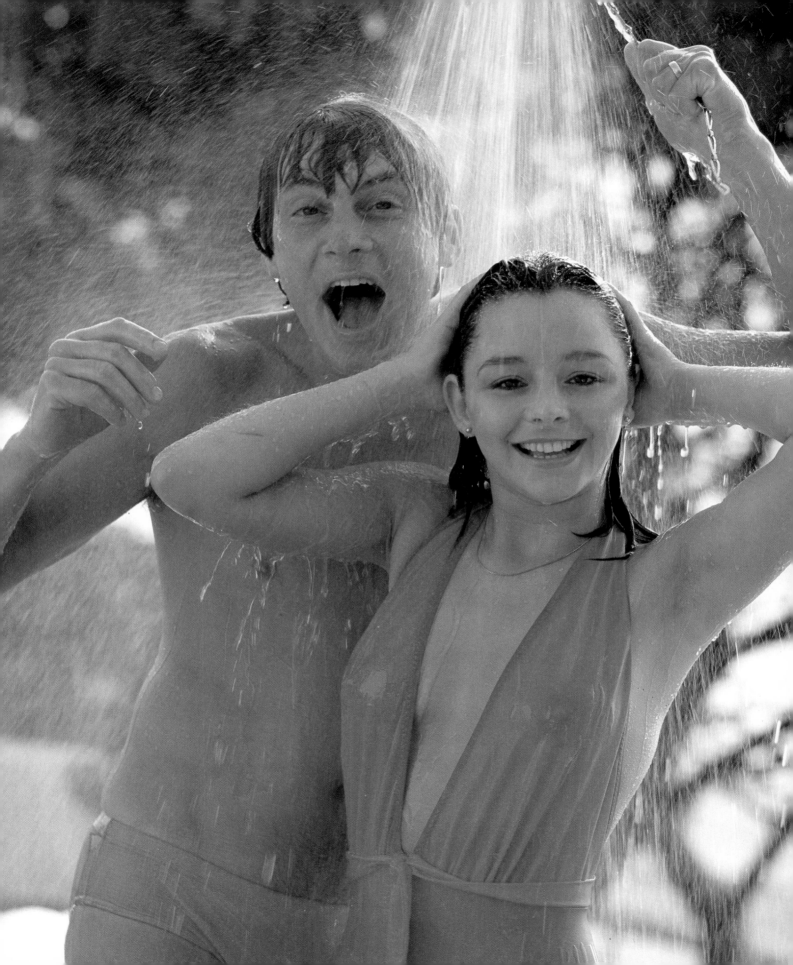

Opposite: we know now that a child's health can be affected by the mother's health habits even before she becomes pregnant! There's no greater gift to pass on to children than the habit of eating well, taking exercise, good posture, deep breathing and knowing how to relax.

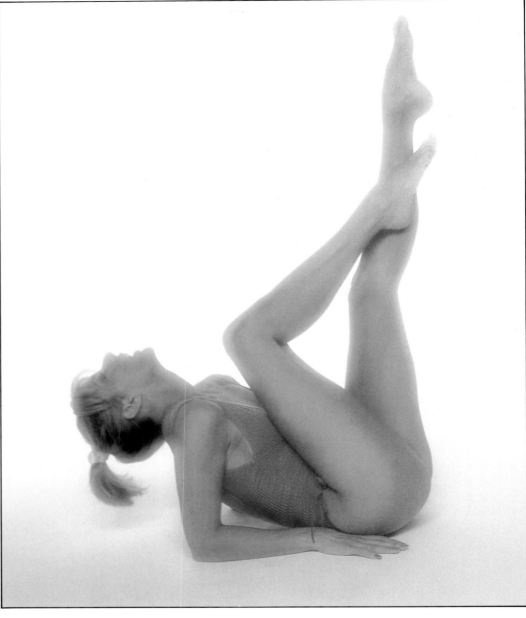

Right: feeling 'good in your skin' isn't a pleasure reserved for the young and perfectly shaped. You can revel in feeling well and in shape at any age: it's never too early – or too late – to start.

but it's also hugely influenced by health. You know for yourself how your own looks suffer when you're feeling unwell. Building up your health builds up your potential for looking great. Without good health, it doesn't matter how wonderful your features are: your eyes won't shine, your skin won't bloom, your hair won't gleam, and you're not likely to have a lovely smile, either.

Today's style of beauty is more closely tied to a healthy vitality than ever before. Once upon a time, models may have wanted to look pale and interesting; now they'd just look anaemic. Heavy make-up is out and, anyway, the one effect it can't produce is that of glowing health.

Feeling really chock full of health is good for your mood, too. It's not surprising that you are more cheerful when you're full of energy and in shape. That 'glow' is essential to today's kind of good looks, as well as making life much more fun.

Deciding to live in a healthier way is like stepping on to an upwards spiral staircase. Choosing food that does more for you and taking exercise don't just improve your level of health by staving off illness, they also give you a good mental feeling that you're looking after yourself and that you are someone worth looking after.

As your body improves – healthy food happens to be the kind that does most for your figure, skin and hair – your confidence

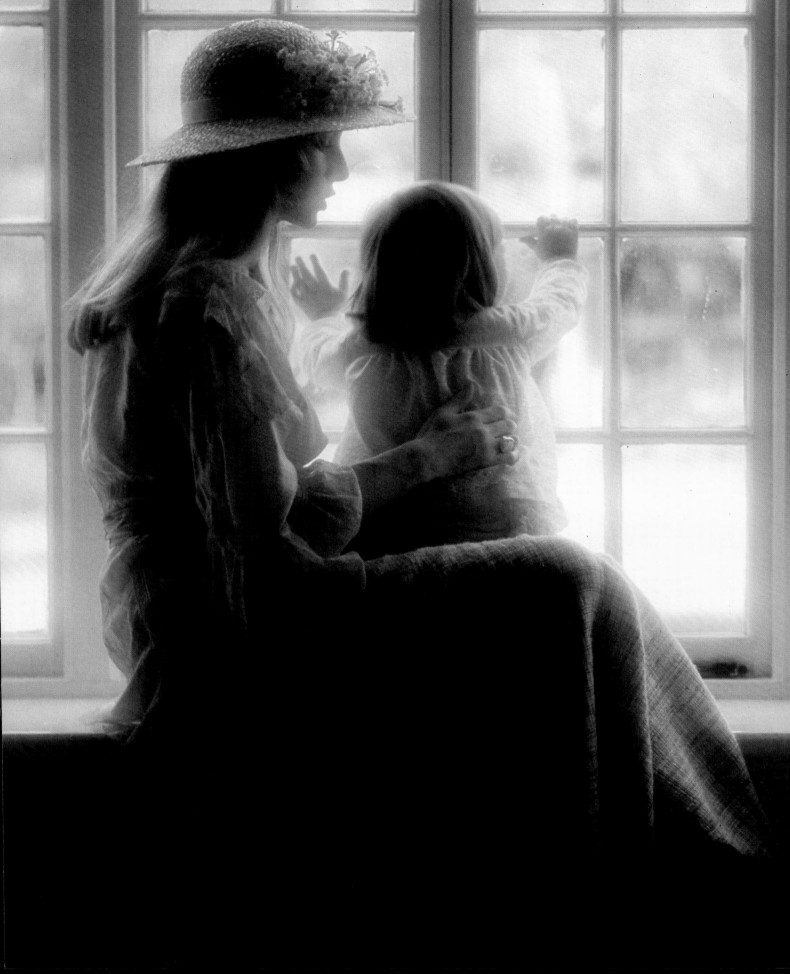

goes up. That helps you in social and professional life, and you therefore feel even better.

When you have a good level of self-confidence, which is a mile away from being bigheaded, you find that life's ups and downs are easier to 'ride'. They still happen, but you don't react with large swings in mood nearly so much. You're able to be philosophical, maintain your sense of wellbeing and come out smiling.

So here's the carrot! Good health habits are worth a little effort because they bring quick, as well as long-term rewards:

* You feel good for more of the time.
* You have a better level of energy to put into work and leisure.
* Life looks rosier, thanks to your added stamina and confidence in your looks.
* Robust health may mean better earning potential.
* Your looks improve in a way that make-up and clothes can't achieve.
* You don't need to worry about losing your looks or health early in life.
* Your children may inherit a better constitution.
* You can cope more easily with life's problems.

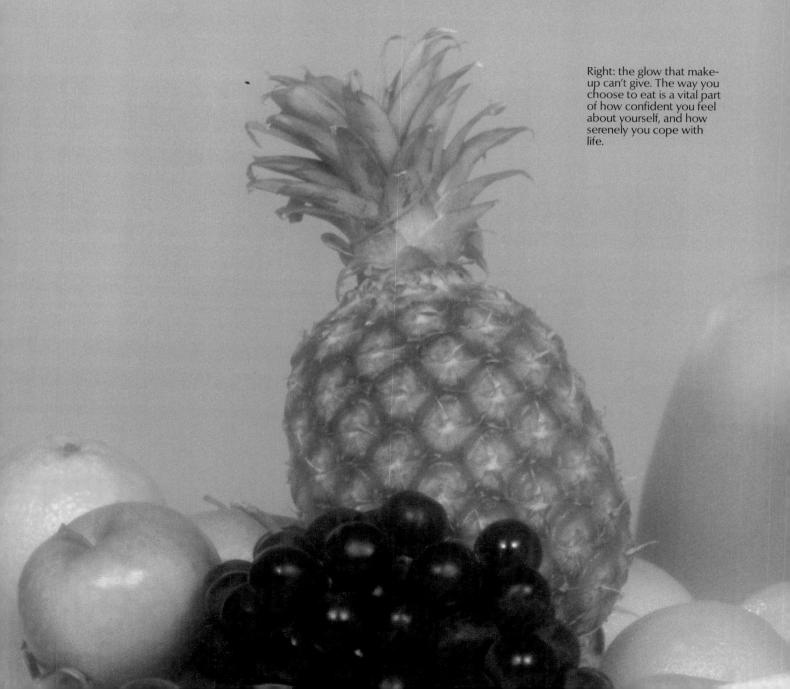

Right: the glow that make-up can't give. The way you choose to eat is a vital part of how confident you feel about yourself, and how serenely you cope with life.

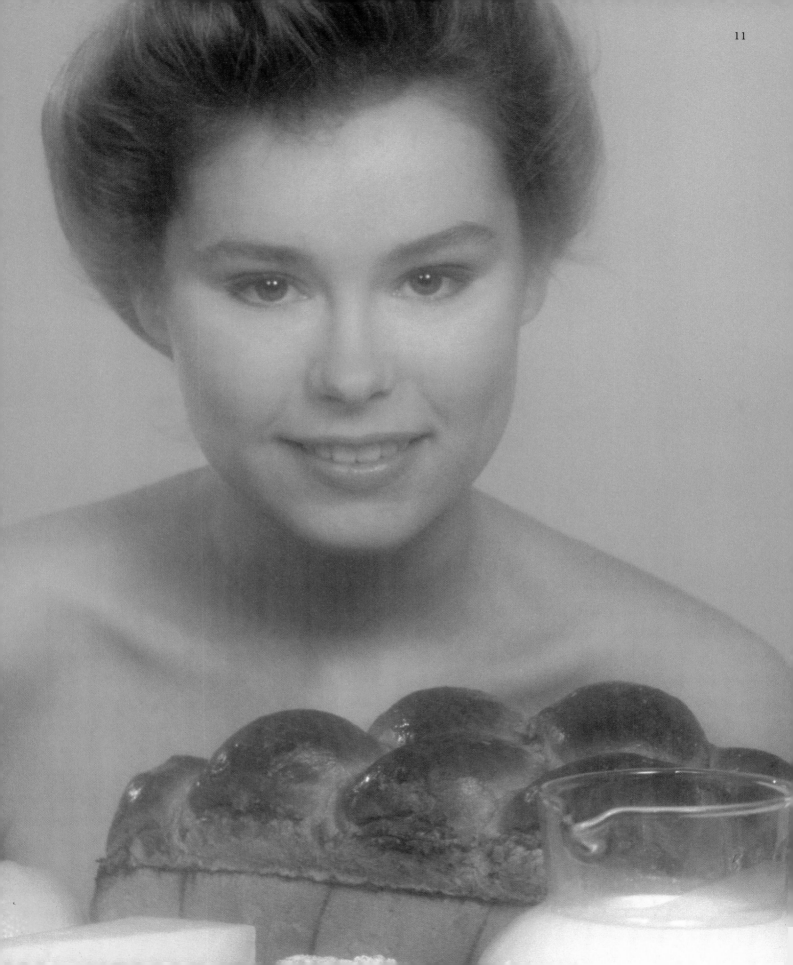

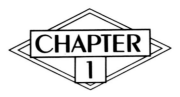

CHAPTER 1

How's the Balancesheet?

A good way to start improving the parts of your life style that affect health is to take a look at what you do now. Here's a check list of factors known to affect your health. It's like playing snakes and ladders; you'll find that some of your regular habits are helping your health without you realising it. Some of the 'snakes' your health can slither down may come as surprises, too. Take a look and be honest with yourself!

effects on health. Women who smoke, for instance, suffer more stillbirths and their babies are more likely to be underweight or die. People who smoke 20 cigarettes a day are twice as likely to die from a heart attack

Opposite: taking 20 minutes to take stock of your living habits, and what they are doing to you, is your best investment.

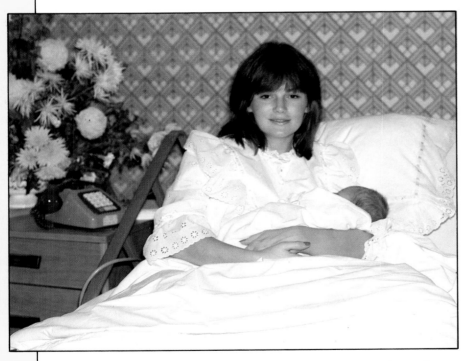

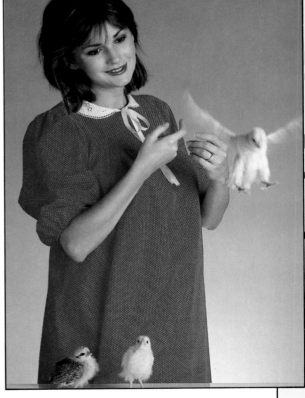

Above: smoking is now seen as taboo for the woman who wants to do the best for her baby – and herself. Much of a baby's health is decided before a woman even knows she is pregnant – so give up before you plan to conceive.

Smoking is your biggest health 'snake'. It isn't just that one in eight of those who smoke over 20 a day will get lung cancer. It's also that smoking is linked with an estimated one in three of all cases of cancer, associated with cancer of the lips, tongue, palate, throat and larynx. In men, there's a link between smoking and cancer of the bladder and, perhaps, cancer of the prostate gland, too.

Most smokers won't get cancer, but there's little chance of escaping its other

as non-smokers. Then there's bronchitis and emphysema, both serious lung complaints which can kill you. Bronchitis that is bad enough to need hospital admission is five times more likely for a heavy smoker.

However, forget the long-term hazards for a minute. You may think 'I'll stop before I get old enough for those problems', but any cigarette you smoke is hurting your health in other ways:

✻ It's affecting your stomach. Smokers

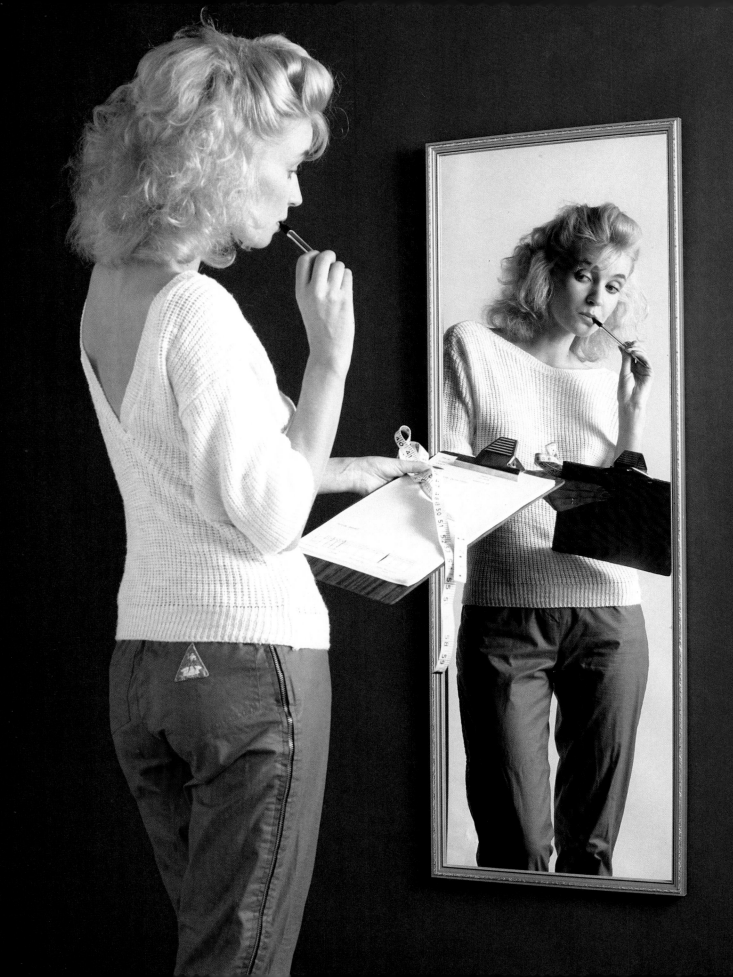

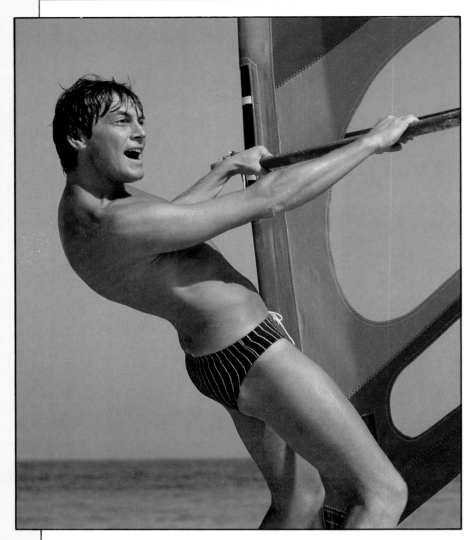

who suffer from heartburn, nausea, flatulence or tummy discomfort often find that stopping solves the problem.

✳ It's affecting your face: smokers tend to screw up their faces as they puff – watch people doing it – and hence get wrinkles more quickly.

✳ It's using up extra vitamin C, reducing your protection against infections.

✳ It's making you smell like an old ashtray. However often you bathe, the smell of tobacco hangs around your breath, your clothes, your home and even your pets and children.

✳ It's putting off other people. Look at how many advertisements for jobs, flat-sharers and mates now specify 'non-smoker'. There are now considerably more non-smokers than smokers and, even if they say nothing, non-smokers may avoid you if you smoke.

✳ It's taking your breath away. Exercise is good for you, but you can't be very good at it while your lungs are struggling with the effects of a drug like nicotine.

✳ It's costing you a small fortune. Even 10 cigarettes a day now costs you the equivalent of a Mediterranean holiday each year.

Smoking and Your Figure With all these reasons to stop, why do almost four out of every ten of us still smoke? Apart from the fact that nicotine is an addictive drug – although that hasn't stopped thousands of people from giving it up – some people may go on smoking because they are frightened to stop; they're worried about putting on weight.

It's true that most people do put on some weight when they stop smoking, but they don't have to stay at that weight. In any case, with care, many avoid gaining even a pound. Although stopping smoking means that your appetite and digestive system get back to normal, so you may feel hungrier and absorb food better, you can counter gaining weight as follows:

✳ Put a temporary 'stop' on alcohol at the same time. Smokers tend to drink more and alcohol has lots of calories. If you stop drinking those calories for a month or two after smoking, you'll reduce your chances of gaining weight, without losing any vitamins or minerals for which alcohol is pretty useless.

✳ Take up an extra form of exercise at the same time. The cash you save on tobacco can pay for an exercise class, for instance. So you'll be using up the extra calories, as well as keeping your mind off the urge to

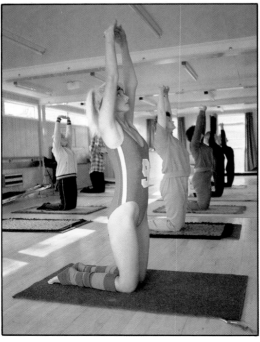

Exercise can help you stop smoking – by giving you something else to do, by providing the relaxation that you may try to get by smoking, and by strengthening your will-power as you find how much not smoking helps your breathing and muscles.

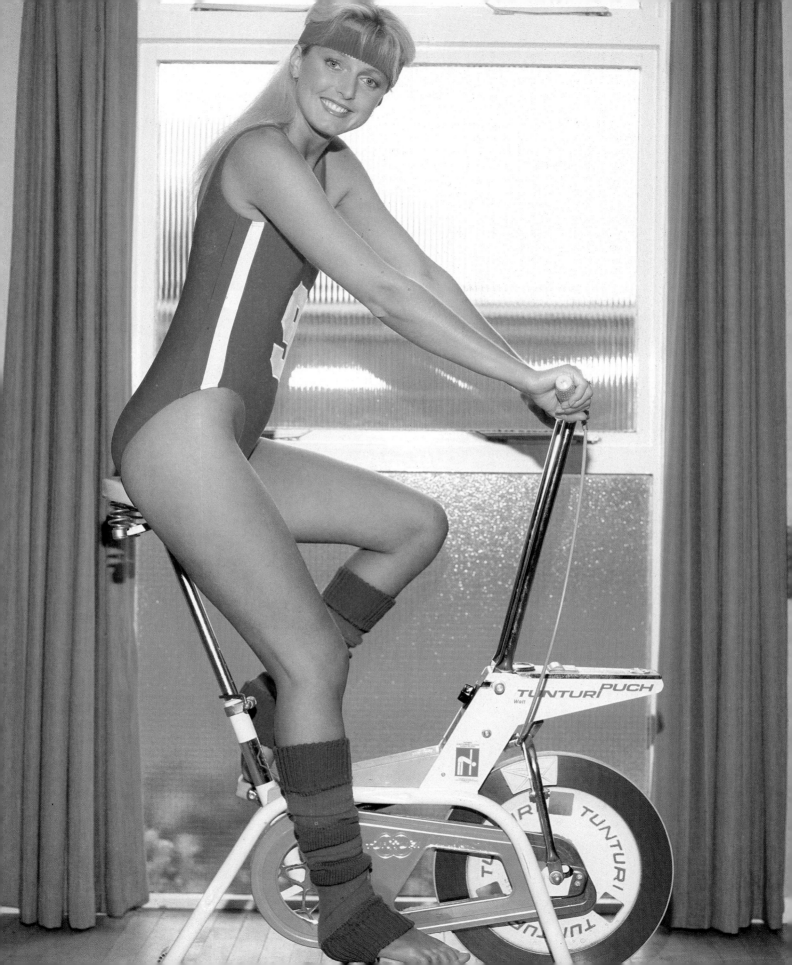

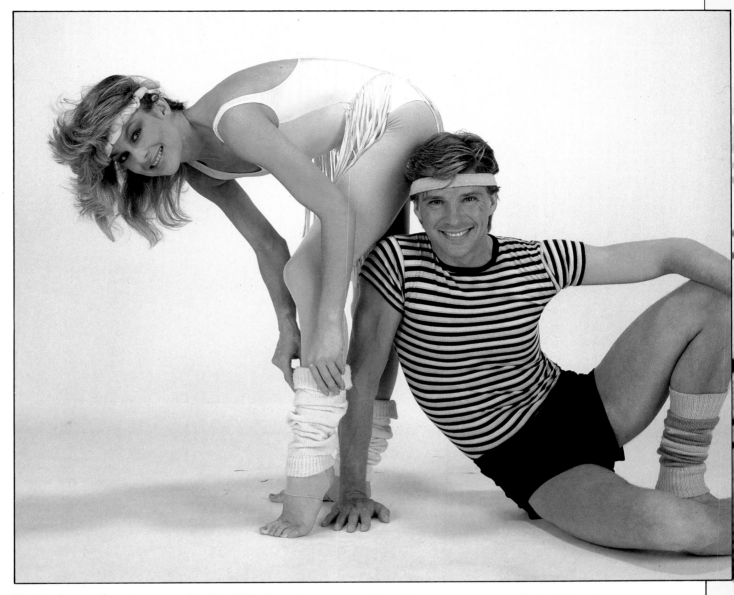

Exercise does not have to hurt, in fact it shouldn't. Push, don't jerk – and don't be put off by your limitations. You'll still feel good – and look better – for each session.

smoke. You'll find you have more 'breath', once you stop smoking, for dancing or just running for a bus.

✳ Change to healthier food at the same time. As you'll find later in the book, it tends to give you more to eat without more calories, so you always have something to chew instead of smoking that cigarette.

Exercise is a good 'ladder' which you may already be using. Whether you have an energetic job, such as teaching swimming, or a regular active sport, if you are taking vigorous exercise three or more times a week, you've got a head start for health.

For many people, exercise is mainly a way of improving the figure. It certainly does that by toning up muscles and using up calories, so you end up in better shape. However, exercise does even more. It

improves circulation, bringing more oxygen to every cell and so promoting alertness and good body function. It strengthens the internal 'slings' which hold your organs in place, so they are able to work well, and it improves your heart and lung efficiency. It is also one of the best ways of relaxing, partly because it takes your mind off anxieties – you can't think of anything but what you are physically concentrating on and, when you come back to your usual 'grind', you get a fresher view – and partly because energetic exercise stimulates the production of mood-raising chemicals in the body.

A 'sitting-still' job is a small 'snake' we can offset by exercise. However, make sure you aren't increasing its chance of affecting your health by one of the following habits:

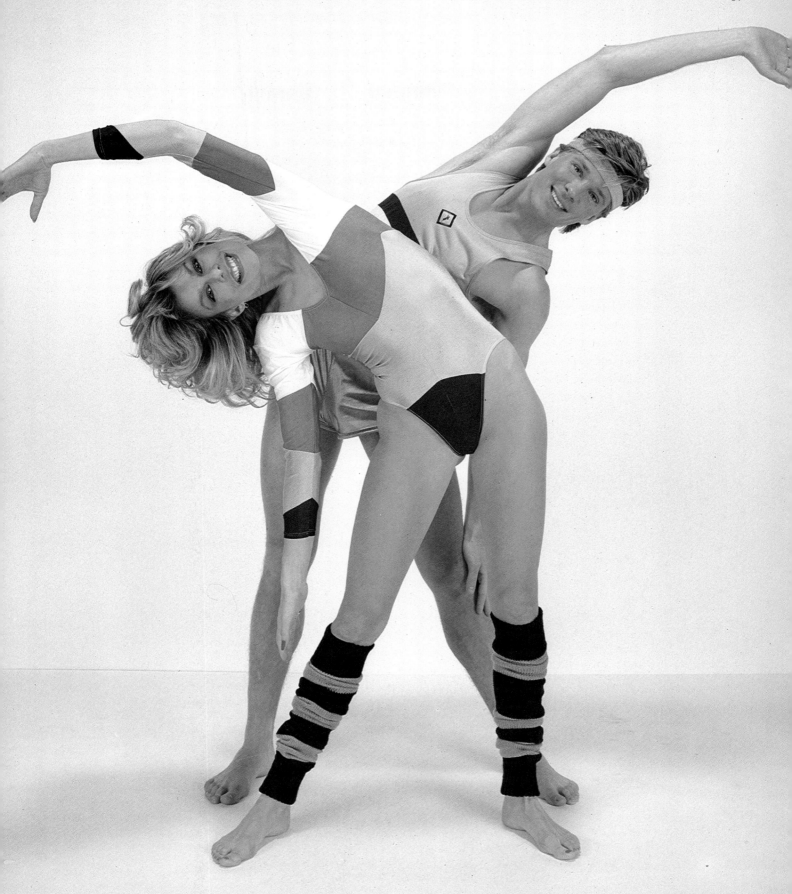

How's the Balancesheet?

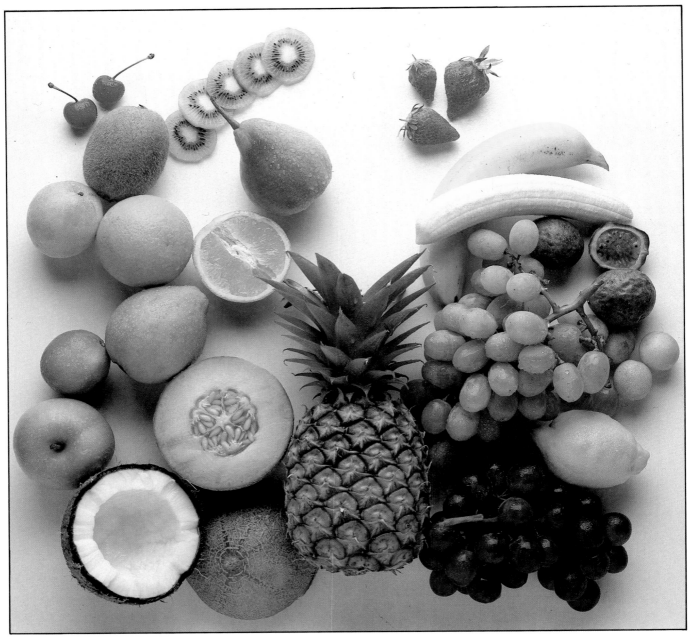

The wonderful world of fruit and vegetables. Make a resolution to make the most of their colours, flavours and variety, instead of spending just as much money on fatty, sugary foods.

sitting in a way that constricts your circulation – slumping, having a chair that digs into the back of your legs, constantly crossing one knee over the other or twisting your back because your chair doesn't fit your needs – or downing cup after cup of tea or coffee and perhaps lots of 'nibbles', too. Even if you don't take sugar or have a packet of peppermints handy, the amount of caffeine in several cups of either tea or coffee can leave you feeling nervy and your system overstimulated.

Eating plenty of fruit and vegetables is a good ladder to health because they provide the least processed form of

vitamins and minerals, and are full of useful fibre in a low-calorie form.

Fruit is useful for minerals and yellow fruit, like apricots, yellow melons, peaches or bananas, provide sources of vitamin A. However, the main advantage of fruit is that its sweetness keeps us away from unhealthy sticky buns and sweets, and it's also a way of getting vitamin C. We all know that citrus fruit, like an orange, is high in vitamin C. However, remember that the level in strawberries is even higher and other soft fruits – particularly the famous blackcurrants, which are one of the highest sources of all – combine vitamin C with a particularly high amount of fibre.

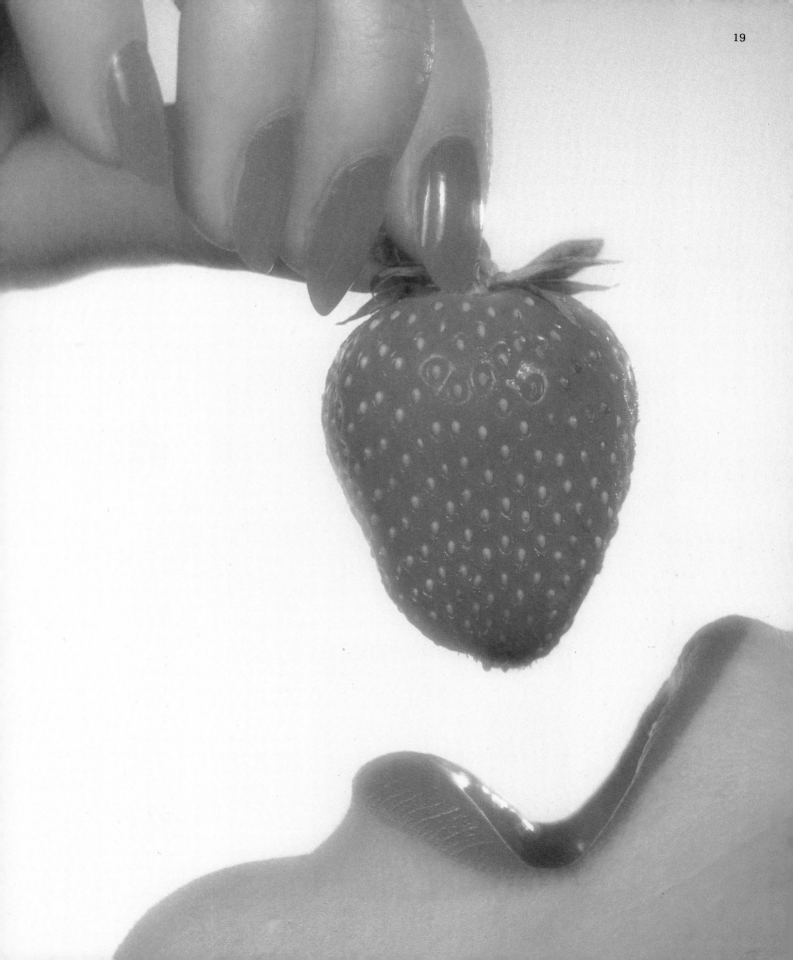

How's the Balancesheet?

Opposite: do you need a 'carrot' to encourage you to change to healthier eating? If health doesn't seem a big enough reward, how about that sheen of healthy good looks!

Of course, you'll only be getting all this good value if you eat fruit fresh or freshly cooked with the juice. Fruit that's been chopped into a fruit salad hours ago and is browning at the edges, or that's tinned in heavy sugar syrup, has already lost a large amount of its nutritional value and gained unwanted sugar, which doesn't have vitamins or minerals.

Some people never eat fruit but stay healthy because they eat vegetables, which are really more important. As well as providing vitamin C and A – again, mainly in yellow or red items like carrots and tomatoes, but also in leafy greens – vegetables provide the main source of other vitamins: the B vitamin folic acid, vitamin E and vitamin K. They also contain

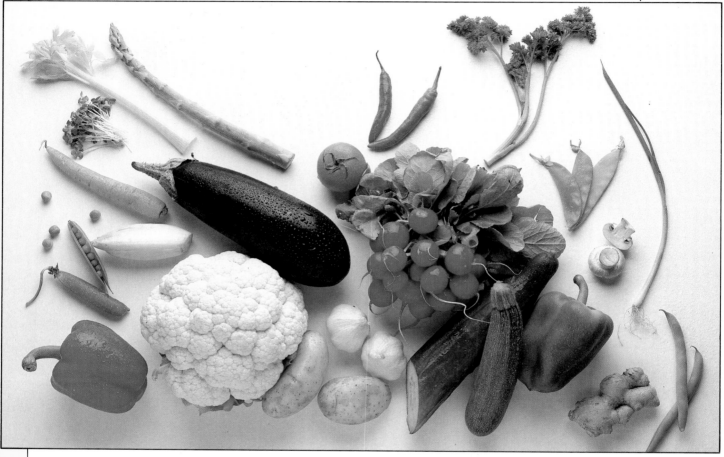

Above and right: vegetables – fresh, leafy, crunchy and colourful – can be your daily health 'insurance'. The more you eat raw, the better – try thinly sliced courgettes, mushrooms, green beans and peas, as well as familiar celery and carrots, for your meals and the snacks that help keep you away from chocolate bars.

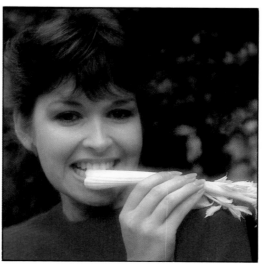

calcium, iron, magnesium and other useful minerals. Green, leafy vegetables are the best for promoting health. So anyone who regularly buys watercress, mustard and cress, spring greens or Chinese leaves, for instance, has a health habit worth cherishing.

Overeating is a 'snake' most of us know well, because it shows, but it doesn't just mean eating too much. It also refers to the kind of food that you eat. Basically, fat and sugar provide a lot of calories in even a small amount of food. Weigh out for yourself an ounce of butter or margarine, and it's astonishing to realise that this little lump contains 10 per cent of all the calories an average woman would eat in a day. Weigh out an ounce of sugar, about 4

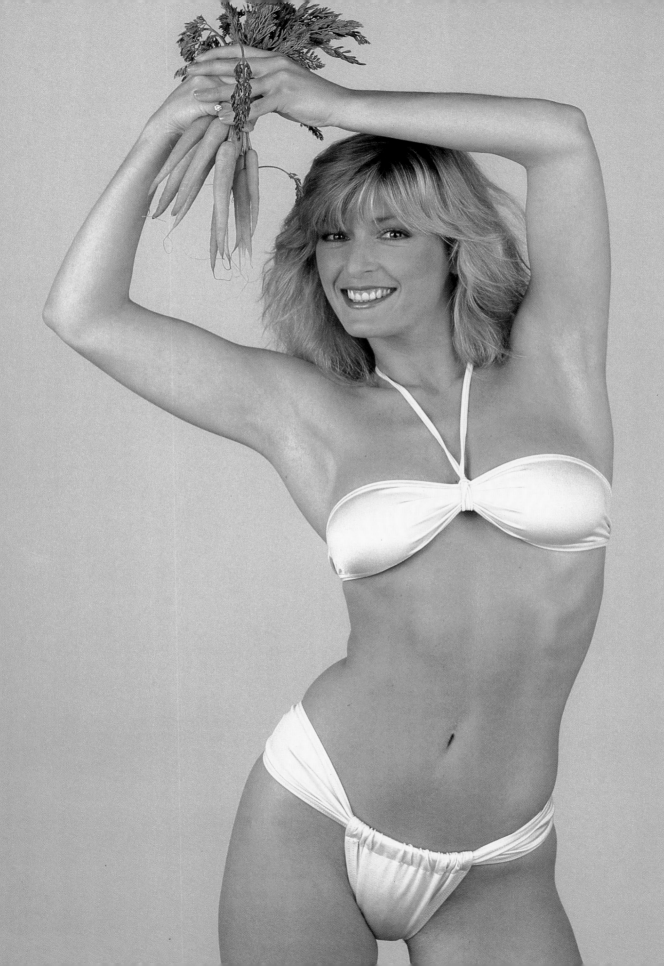

teaspoonfuls, and it's the same story.

Because most of us have to eat a certain amount of food to feel full, any dish that includes a lot of these high-calorie-for-their-bulk foods is likely to end up consuming a very large amount of calories. Calories aren't 'bad' – they're the energy input we need to keep us alive and kicking – but if we eat more than we use up in energy, we store those calories as fat.

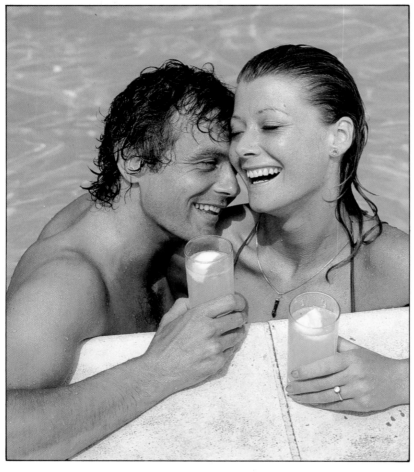

Above and opposite: sugar *isn't* needed for exercise – or romance! But soft drinks and alcohol such as sweeter wines can hide a lot. Try 'drier' drinks – like fruit juice or dry wine, mixed half-and-half with sparkling mineral water.

We all know someone who seems to be able to eat any amount of rich, sugary foods without gaining weight. These people react to extra food, it seems, by turning up their body 'thermostat', so that the surplus is burnt off. However, few people can do that permanently if they keep swallowing too many calories. By the time they are thirty years old, the extra starts to show on many a previously slender frame. Also, those who stay permanently hungry and thin are likely to be nervous, highly strung individuals; so we shouldn't envy them too much.

The fact remains that meals with lots of sugar or fat are deceptively high in calories, and we can overeat even if we don't seem to eat large platefuls. In contrast, if you choose food that's low in fat and sugar, you can eat much more and feel fuller, and still end up with fewer calories. Here's where healthy eating shows its double benefit. Reducing the amount of fat and sugar you eat tends to help you control your weight without having to think about it all the time, and it also helps your general health.

Sugar is the only food we eat that contains none of the 40-plus vitamins and minerals we need for good health. It's often described as 'empty calories'. So cutting out sugar, and you don't *need* crystal sugar for energy or for any other purpose, saves a lot of calories – 110 per ounce – which you can 'spend' on more nourishing foods. Anything else you eat instead, apart from fat, will provide some of the nourishment you need. With the average person consuming one in five of all their calories through sugar, in food, drinks and alcohol, that's a lot of extra goodness you can get by eating other foods instead. Usually this means fewer calories too, as other foods are more filling.

Fat isn't 'empty calories' and you shouldn't try a 'fat-free diet' because you need some fat to stay healthy. On the other hand, most people eat around four out of every ten calories in the form of fat. That's around twice as much fat as we need for good health. The surplus half merely provides a whopping amount of calories: 205 per ounce for butter or margarine, 255 for oil. So reducing fat saves you more calories than reducing any other food, but you lose less volume off your plate, because fat is so compact.

Eating too much fat or sugar hurts your health prospects in other ways; you'll read later in this book how. For the moment, however, just keep in mind that if you eat 1oz less sugar and 1oz less fat each day – most of us down about 3-4oz of each – that's at least 315 calories you can either spend on more nutritious foods, or save in a diet. A pound of unwanted flesh comprises some 3,500 surplus calories, and 315 saved calories daily adds up to around 32½lb a year less you! You'll probably use some of those calories on other foods but, even so, it's the easiest way to keep your weight under control without thinking about it.

Overeating may be a 'snake' for you because you eat too much fat and sugar, therefore too many calories, or because you go on eating and eating even when you know you aren't hungry. Compulsive eating is so common, it's nothing to be ashamed of or to hide. Lots of people around you do

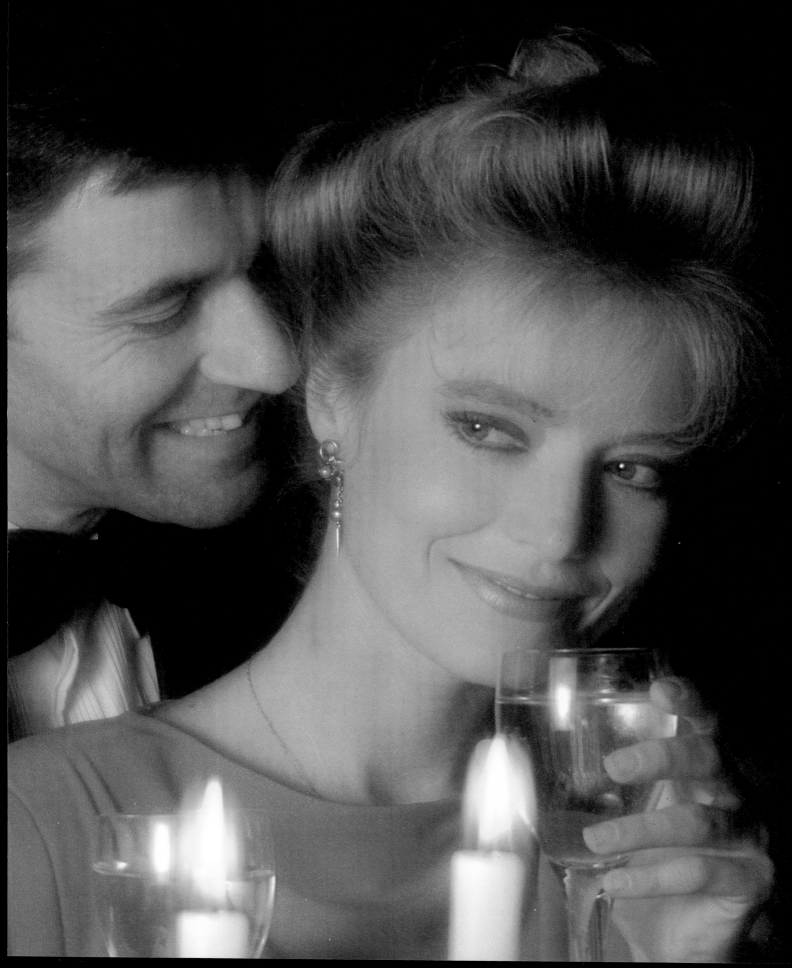

Opposite and below: you don't need a leotard to benefit from exercise and active hobbies. Here are two that make life fun. Gardening and riding can be energetic, or just absorbing. Either way, they'll relax you by giving your mind a refreshing break from tension and worries, in the fresh air.

it, but some do it more than others. If you find yourself turning to food – especially chocolate, cakes and other sweet and gooey foods – when you're upset, angry, bored, worried or fed up with your life, cutting down fat and sugar isn't the answer for you. You won't to able to, unless you tackle the troubled state of mind behind the urge to 'binge'.

Relaxation can help as you will see later in this book. As one of the most difficult things is admitting the seething emotions underneath those cream cakes, you may need to find someone you can 'let it all out' to, such as a professional counsellor or a self-help group of other overeaters who understand and can offer their success stories to give you hope of getting out of the cream pit!

Hobbies that keep you interested and on the move are another 'ladder'. Energetic ones, such as running a playgroup or gardening, are the most useful but anything that you're really keen on has a health value. That's because it puts you in a good mood, enhances your confidence in yourself as a capable and useful person, and absorbs the energy you might otherwise spend on worrying, feeling bored, frustrated, or depressed at the apparent emptiness of your life.

There's little doubt that feeling miserable is bad for you. We take for granted such sayings as 'bored to tears', 'painfully lonely' or, when angry, 'it makes me sick', but they reflect the way that our emotions can make us feel ill and even reduce our resistance to infection. Studies of American students

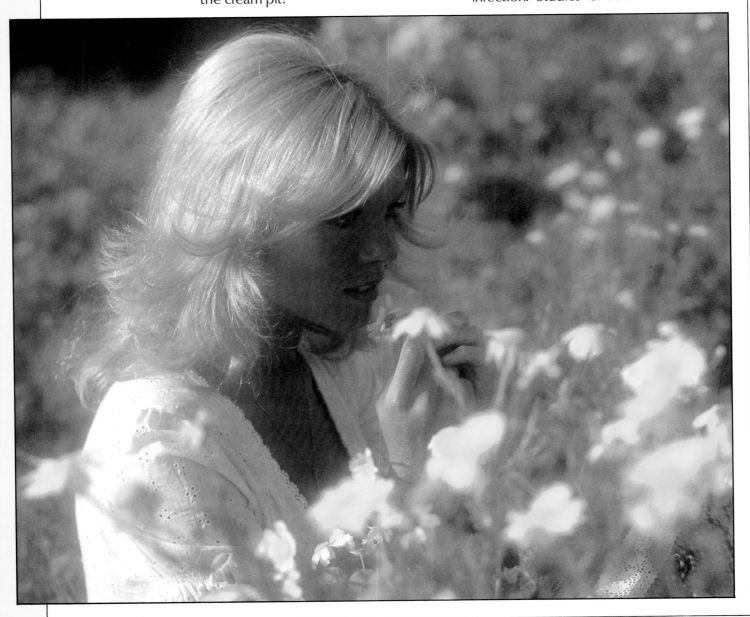

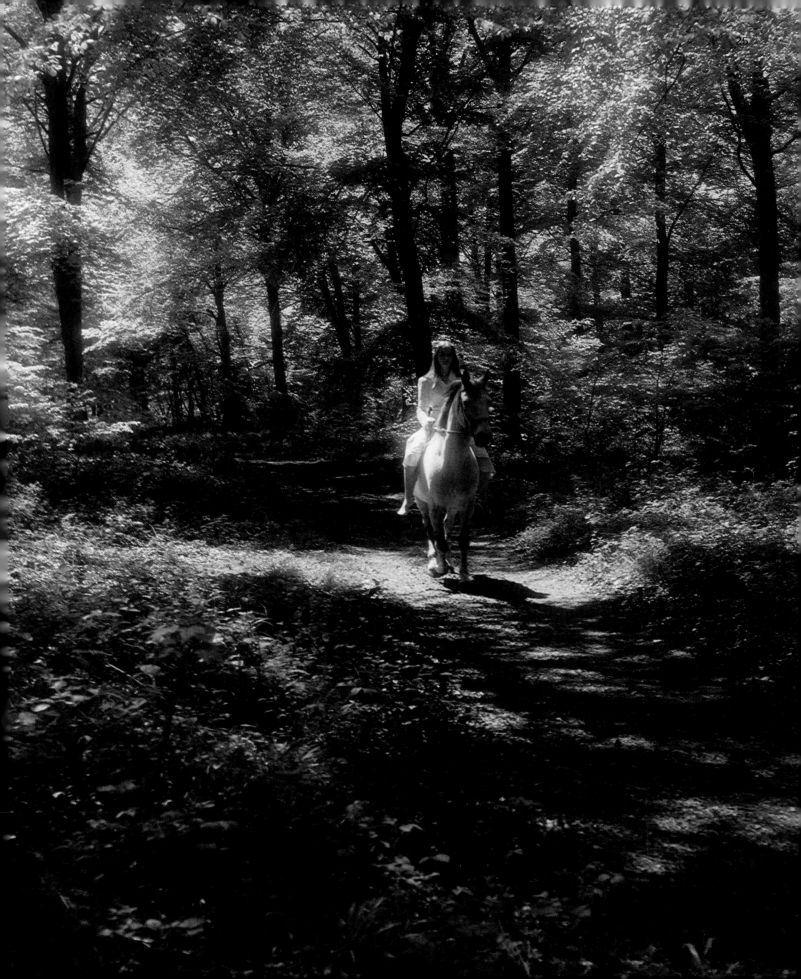

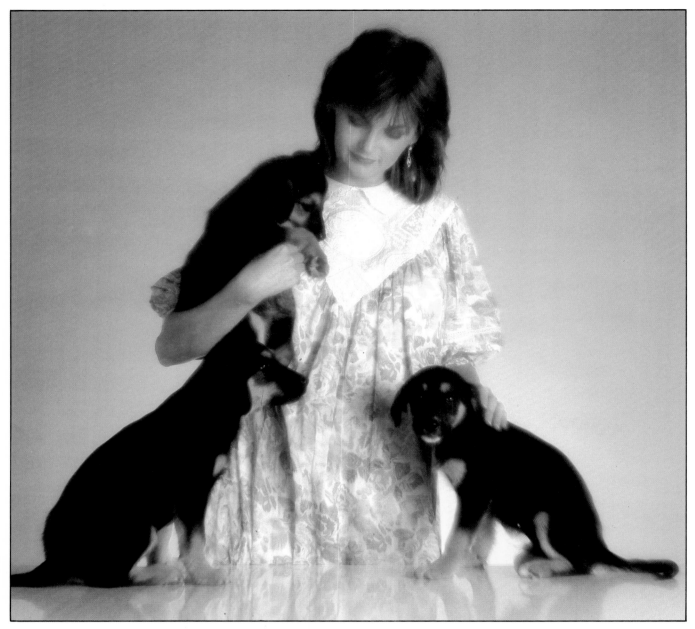

Above and opposite: when you are absorbed in a hobby where you acquire knowledge and skill, your confidence, together with your ability to cope with stress, will benefit.

have shown, for example, that at the times of year when they were most worried about examinations, their body's defence system against infection worked far less efficiently.

A sense of self-value is important to all of us in day-to-day self-confidence and also in making us feel less depressed when life goes wrong. One of the best ways of gaining a permanent improvement in how you see yourself is to develop a skill. It doesn't really matter what it is: stamp-collecting, flower-arranging, card tricks, folk songs or growing azaleas. What's important is to know that you are unusually knowledgeable and skilled in at least one area of life; something of which you can

remind yourself when you doubt your abilities in other fields. With shorter hours spent in work inside or outside the home, there's more opportunity than ever to develop such a skill and more people eager to teach it in evening classes or clubs.

Too much alcohol is a 'snake' that can easily get out of hand. While the odd glass of wine or beer doesn't seem to harm people, the number of those whose lives are dominated by their addiction to alcohol is rising, particularly among women. The increase may be due to a mixture of influences and it's interesting to look hard at one's own drinking pattern to see how and why one drinks. It's more

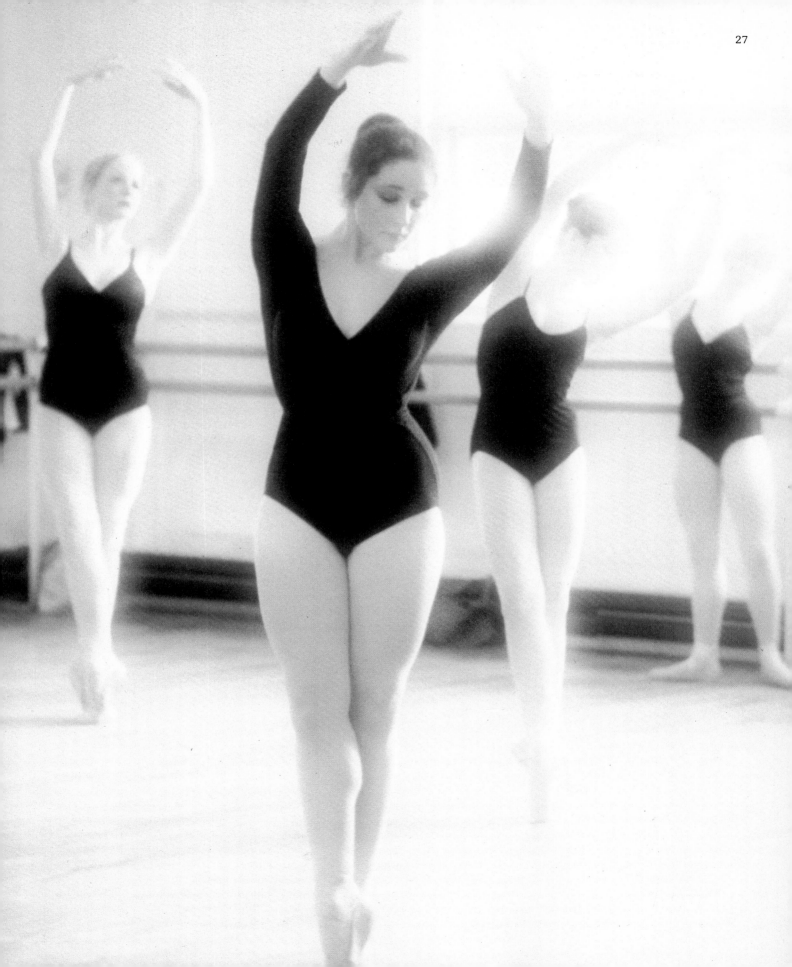

acceptable for women to drink than it used to be and young people still see getting drunk as part of growing up and being sophisticated. Many people have more spare time – some by choice, some not – and drinking can grow to dangerous amounts almost without realising it, through having more hours to socialise.

It's now medically established that women are more at risk from heavy drinking than men, suffering from liver damage more easily. Also, drinking in pregnancy affects babies badly and, unfortunately, by the time a woman knows she's pregnant, the baby has usually been developing for several weeks. The alcohol drunk during that period can already have given it a setback, for the very early weeks of pregnancy are the time of fastest brain development for the foetus. Today, the advice to women is that if you plan to have a baby, or even know you're liable to accidents, don't drink, or limit it to a maximum of a glass a day.

Alcohol is bad for your figure in two ways. Firstly, it's got a surprising number of calories. Secondly, it's spoiled many a diet by relaxing the willpower of the dieter, so that after a glass of wine the person concerned tucks into the gateaux or peanuts.

Like sugar, alcohol is 'empty calories', so omitting it can only help. If you eat more of other things with the saved calories, you're bound to get more goodness out of them than you would out of the alcohol, without the bleary eyes, headache and bags under your eyes!

Alcohol isn't good for mental health, either. Beyond a modest amount, people become aware that they aren't fully in control – an uncomfortable feeling – and they also feel weak-willed, losing self-respect. The idea that hard drinking is somehow 'strong' is losing ground and, while a small amount of alcohol is a stimulant, what goes up comes down with a thump: it's really a depressant in any quantity.

Not being a rusher is a help up the ladder of health. People who are not always trying to fit too much into their time make far less tension for themselves; they aren't constantly struggling to keep up with their tight schedule, worrying about the clock or cutting short their personal relationships because they're rushing off elsewhere.

Tension doesn't just take the enjoyment out of life. It also affects your health. Mental tension produces physical tightening of

muscles; feel how tight the back of your neck gets when you are worried, for instance. Prolonged tension, if you don't take time to relax, can produce all kinds of backache, headache and other ills. Your chest muscles will tighten too, restricting how deeply you breathe. One of the first reactions in a tense situation is to start breathing shallowly. It doesn't matter for a short while, but the habit can set in, precipitating asthma attacks and headaches, as well as limiting the supply of oxygen to your body.

Do you remember how it feels when you're stuck in a traffic jam or a delayed train and you know you're going to be late for an important appointment or plane? If your memory is accurate, it will recall that churning of the stomach and possibly even the feeling that you couldn't breathe properly or felt sick. Day-to-day tension may not be so extreme, but it can certainly divert your body from digesting food properly. The result that's best known is ulcers but feeling bloated, and attacks of heartburn and indigestion, are bad enough.

Being in a rush is almost certain to mean that you eat less good food. You'll be more inclined to grab a take-away or open a bar of chocolate, just because it's quick. Unfortunately, both are full of excess fat, sugar and additives; well, not quite all, as you'll see later. It is possible to eat 'fast food' that's good for you, but you have to make a little more effort. If you don't, you may gradually run your system down by not supplying it with the vitamins and minerals you need, especially since stress results in more B group vitamins and vitamin C being used up.

Drinking too much tea, coffee, cola drinks or chocolate is a habit that often goes hand in hand with the person who is always rushing and under stress; it isn't an accident. Unconsciously, most of us are attracted to all four because they contain chemicals which are stimulants; mild stimulants, but strong enough for the person who drinks cup after cup, or eats bar after bar of chocolate, to find it hard to stop. They all contain caffeine and related stimulants which, in excess, make you feel jumpy, 'hepped up' and incapable of sleeping or even slowing down. They affect your digestive as well as nervous systems and, if you give your body a chance to see what it feels like without them, you'll usually find that after a few weeks in which you really miss coffee, suffer from headaches and, perhaps, constipation,

Opposite: don't let life turn into a race against the clock. It will create unnecessary tension, which can lead to headaches, stomach problems, backache and more. You *don't* have to rush: learn to say 'no' charmingly!

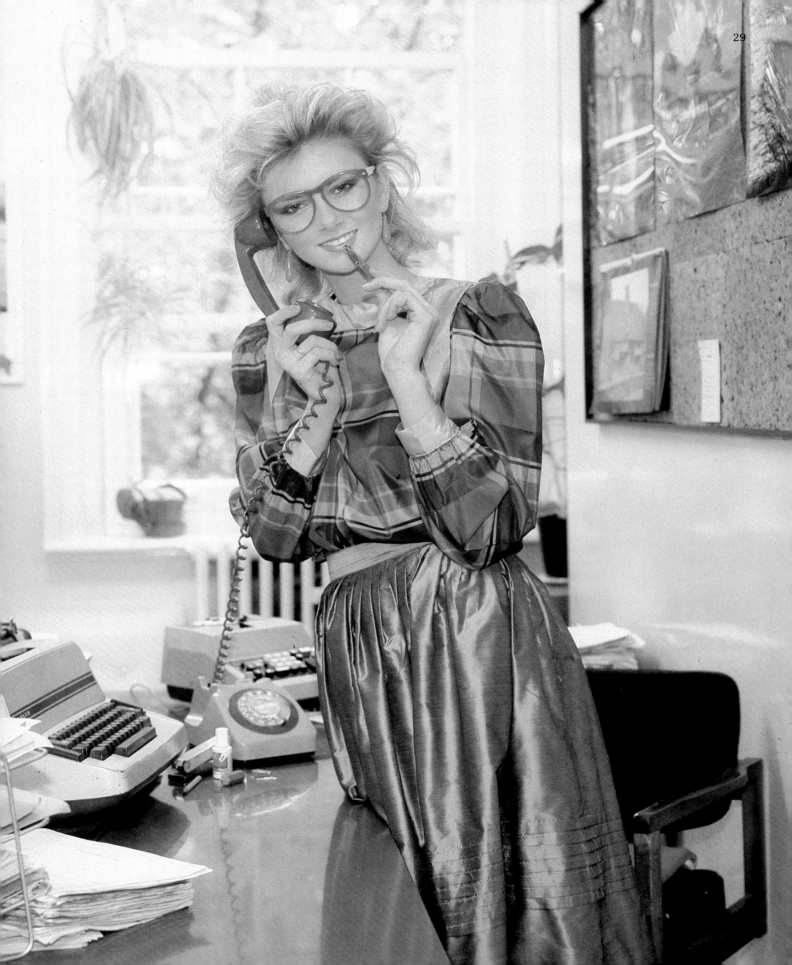

How's the Balancesheet?

Below: eat well during the day (packed meals and snacks can help) and less at night, for fewer weight and health battles. Opposite: buy new toothbrushes regularly, as regular brushing fights tooth-destroying gum disease.

you'll feel far calmer and more in control of your life.

Late night eating is yet another 'snake' which modern life encourages by its rush through each day. It's almost standard to skip breakfast, except for a quick cuppa; pick up a sandwich and cake for lunch to fit round shopping or socialising, and come home ravenous. By the time dinner is cooked, it may be so late that you only have an hour or two before bed. Your digestive system takes longer than that, so it may keep you awake with its gurgles as it tackles the big meal you've enjoyed after eating little all day. Next morning, it's not surprising if you don't feel like breakfast; your digestive system has barely recovered from the night before. The meal you eat late at night is less likely to be used up in activity, especially as your system of burning calories slows down when you sleep. So those calories are more likely to be stored as fat. Your sleep and your digestive system are both suffering if you overload the evening meal.

A study in America, detailed in *The Body Clock Diet* by Ronald Gatty, showed how eating the same number of calories per day, but all in the morning, produced steady weight loss in a group of volunteers, even though they ate just as much. You wouldn't want to go to such extremes, but the principle is worth remembering.

Skipping breakfast isn't a help in slimming; it's much more effective to move some calories from later in the day to breakfast time. If you do so, your evening meal will be lighter and you'll feel hungrier at breakfast, especially if you also try to eat earlier at night.

A settled home life with regular meals is a 'ladder' because it favours healthier eating habits. The more cooking you do at home, the more likely you are to eat plenty of fruit and vegetables, which don't figure highly on restaurant menus and, when they do, have often been overcooked so they've lost a lot of their vitamin C. You're less likely to rely regularly on café fry-ups and take-aways, too.

An old toothbrush is a give-away 'snake' in your bathroom. The main benefit of brushing your teeth well and often is not to brush off sugar and so avoid holes in your teeth; the evidence is that the damage starts very quickly after eating the sugar and that only avoiding its consumption will really make much difference to tooth decay. Tooth brushing's value is in preventing the other 'mouth disease' from which adults lose more teeth than from tooth decay, such as *gingivitis*, or inflammation of the gums from bacterial infection, in which the teeth may become loose in their sockets. The tooth sockets themselves can also become filled with pus, following infection, in the condition *pyorrhoea alveolaris*.

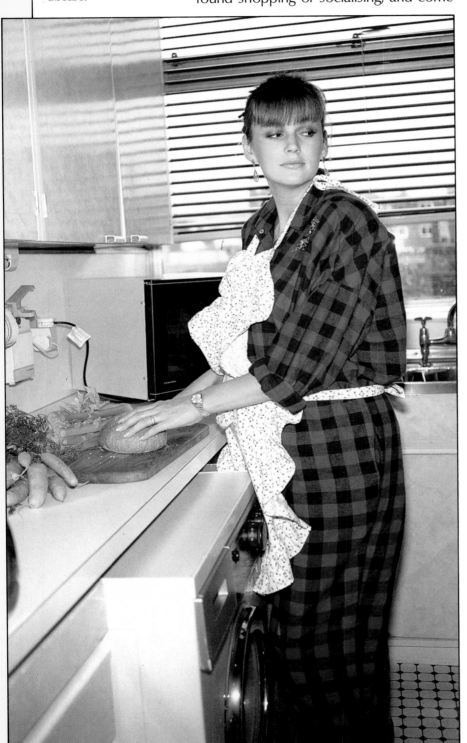

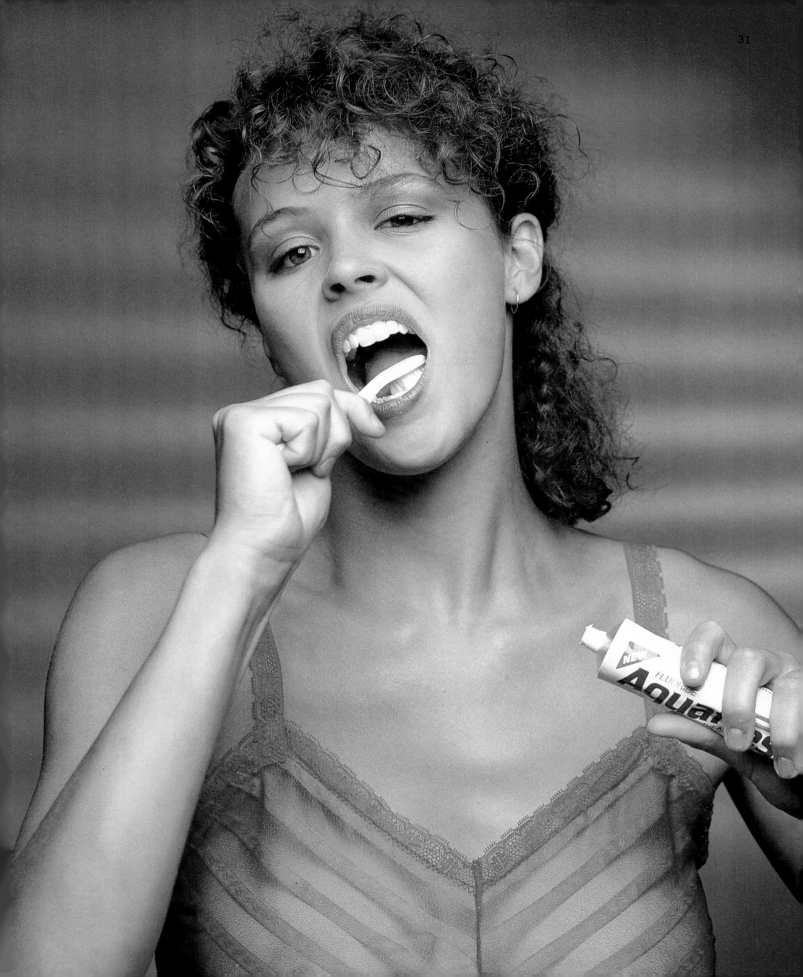

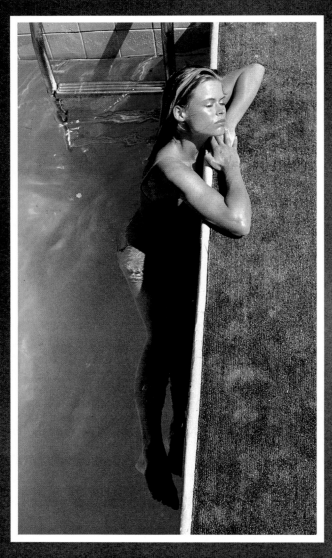

Being good at relaxing is a 'ladder'. Some people are just naturally relaxed; others can learn to be more so by taking up exercise, yoga, meditation or other techniques which show you how to slow down and unwind. Not only does this undo the tension we all experience, which is part of life, so it can't affect our health; it also avoids some of that tension occurring. That's the part that comes not because a train is late, or someone is rude to us, but because we overreact to that upset. You may think that your reactions aren't under your control, but you can almost certainly recall something you got very upset about in the past, which now makes you wonder why. People can learn to take life more philosophically. The first step towards doing so is to become aware of how you react to events and often just watching yourself provides a restraining influence on your emotions!

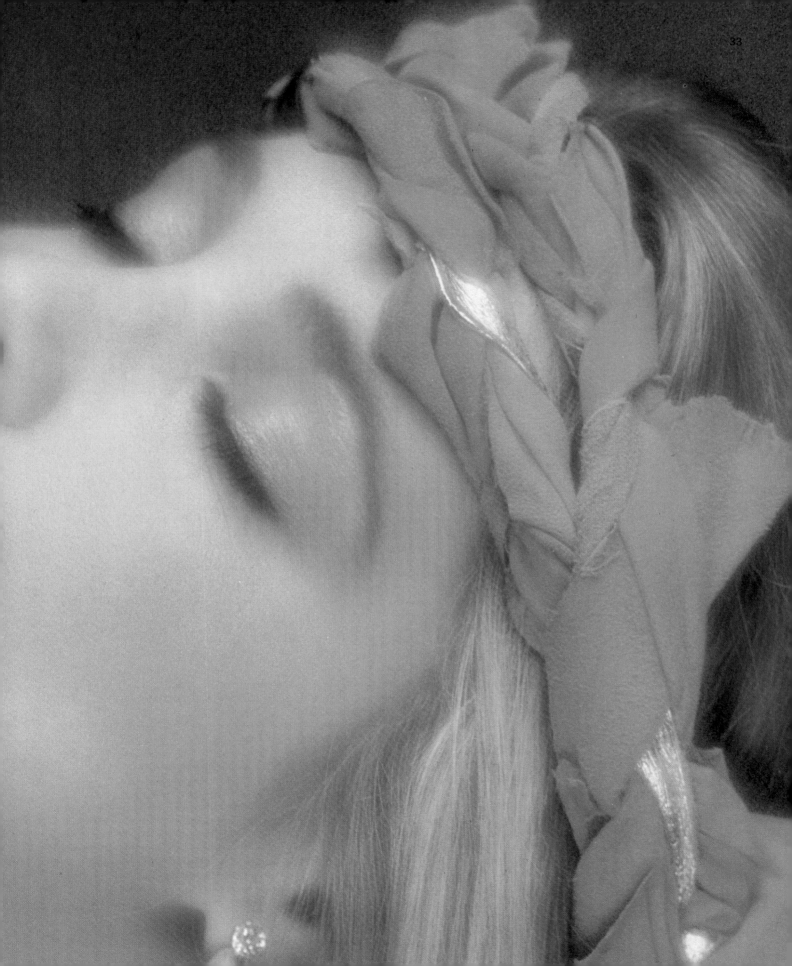

Other Snakes and Ladders

* *Long hours of car driving*, especially if you use your wheels when you could walk, reduce your exercise and can leave you with a stiff back and tension from negotiating heavy traffic.

* *Eating in staff restaurants* or canteens can unbalance your diet through lack of fresh fruit and vegetables, unless you choose carefully.

* *Walking to work*, or at least to the station or bus stop, can give you a surprising amount of exercise, just because you do it so often. A simple way of upping your exercise is to extend this walk by 10 minutes by taking a longer route or walking a few more stops.

* *Having a good laugh now and then* helps your health! When you laugh you relax tense muscles, breathe deeper and put your worries in perspective.

* *Love of cream buns* is more of a psychological hang-up than a real, physical love affair; otherwise, we'd all have the craving! Willpower on its own is a less effective 'cure' than watching yourself to see what emotions spark off the urge. Then transfer them to some non-food, harmless outlet, such as doing a crossword puzzle, buffing your nails, or taking a walk round the block. If you can stave off the urge for 15 to 20 minutes, you'll probably find it's gone; another clue that it's a reaction to emotion, not hunger.

* *Lack of knowledge about healthy eating* is still a major reason why people don't eat better than they do. So now you've had a look at some of the ways you help or hurt your health, here's a closer look at how food can be your ally or your enemy in feeling and looking great.

Lifestyle Quiz

1 *Do you smoke?* A. Never. B. Under 5 a day. C. Over 5 a day.
2 *How often do you eat fresh vegetables or fruit?* A. Daily. B. Weekly. C. An orange at Christmas.
3 *Do you know what your blood pressure is?* A. Yes. B. No idea.
4 *Do you sometimes use sleeping tablets?* A. Yes. B. Never.
5 *Are you happy about your shape, more or less, when you see yourself naked?* A. Ugh! B. Love it! C. Reasonably content.
6 *How many alcoholic drinks do you have a week?* A. Around 1 per day. B. None at all. C. Under 3 a day. D. More, but can't count!
7 *Have you had a health check-up in the last 2 years?* A. Yes. B. No.
8 *Do you consider yourself in general:* A. Relaxed? B. Tense?

Answers

1 Score 0 for A, 2 for B or 6 for C.
2 Score 0 for A, 2 for B or 4 for C.
3 Score 0 for A, 2 for B. It's sensible to have your blood pressure measured from time to time as it's a measure of how hard your heart is having to work to push blood round the body. High blood pressure indicates that your heart is having to work too hard and is a sign of greater risk of heart disease, stroke or kidney problems.
4 Score 3 for A, 0 for B.
5 Score 4 for A, 0 for B, and 0 for C. Liking or being realistically content with your shape – if you're telling the truth – is healthy, suggesting that you've got a reasonably good self-image and confidence, and are in reasonably good shape; not model girl shape but not flabby.
6 Score 0 for A or B, 3 for C and 5 for D. Over 24 drinks a week means you have a drinking problem. Tolerance varies, but many women could be suffering health damage on less. Almost anyone on more than 2 drinks per day would be better off cutting down, both to avoid the excess calories and the heavy workload that alcohol imposes on the liver.
7 Score 0 for A, 2 for B. Check-ups can catch problems while they are still trivial, or show you where your health habits are slipping; for instance, if you find your blood pressure is inching upwards.
8 Score 0 for A and 3 for B. Being a tense person doesn't always bode ill for health – you may just be highly strung like a racehorse – but many people can't cope and develop stress-induced complaints, like stomach problems or skin rashes.

If you've scored:

Over 20: you're fighting your own health! Take action now, before your body rebels.
Over 10: not bad, provided you don't smoke, but wouldn't you like to get even more spring in your step?
0-10: you're heading in the right direction; keep going!

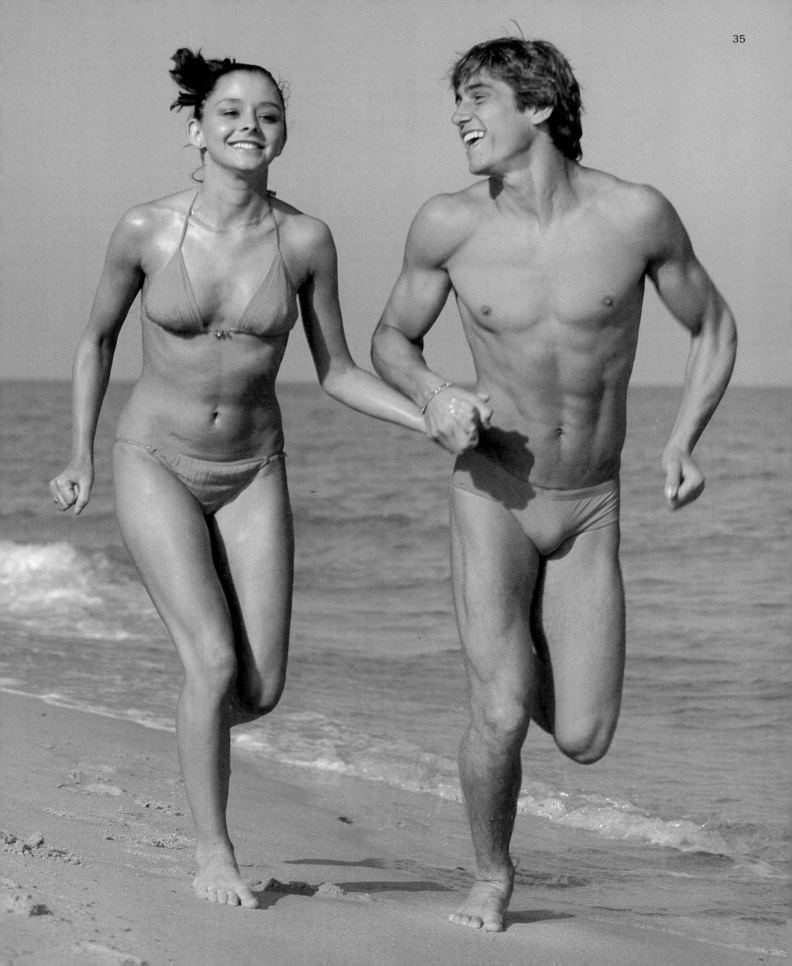

CHAPTER 2

Eating Your way to Health

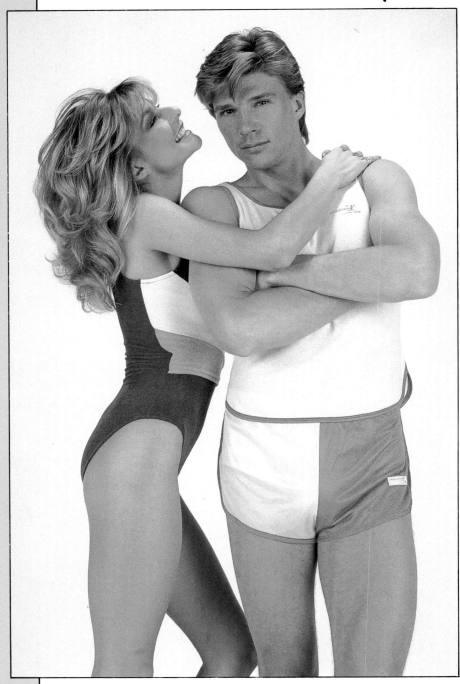

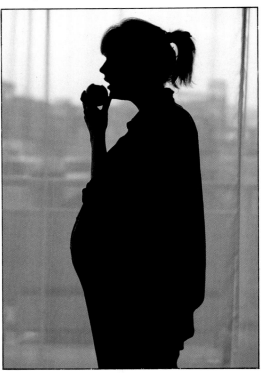

Some people think that eating healthily will turn them into a rabbit: all carrots, lettuce and timidity! Well, it won't. What you eat is one of the most important elements in your health programme, but you don't have to be a fanatic about it, or spend more time, trouble or money. Healthy food can taste good, too.

Some people say that they won't bother about healthy eating because experts disagree so much on what you should eat. Although there's a lot we still don't know about how food affects health, there's enough general agreement, however, to have produced government reports in both the United Kingdom and the United States of America. The advice they've advocated doesn't have to spoil your meals, or make you a social outcast, and it applies just as much to slim people as to fatter ones.

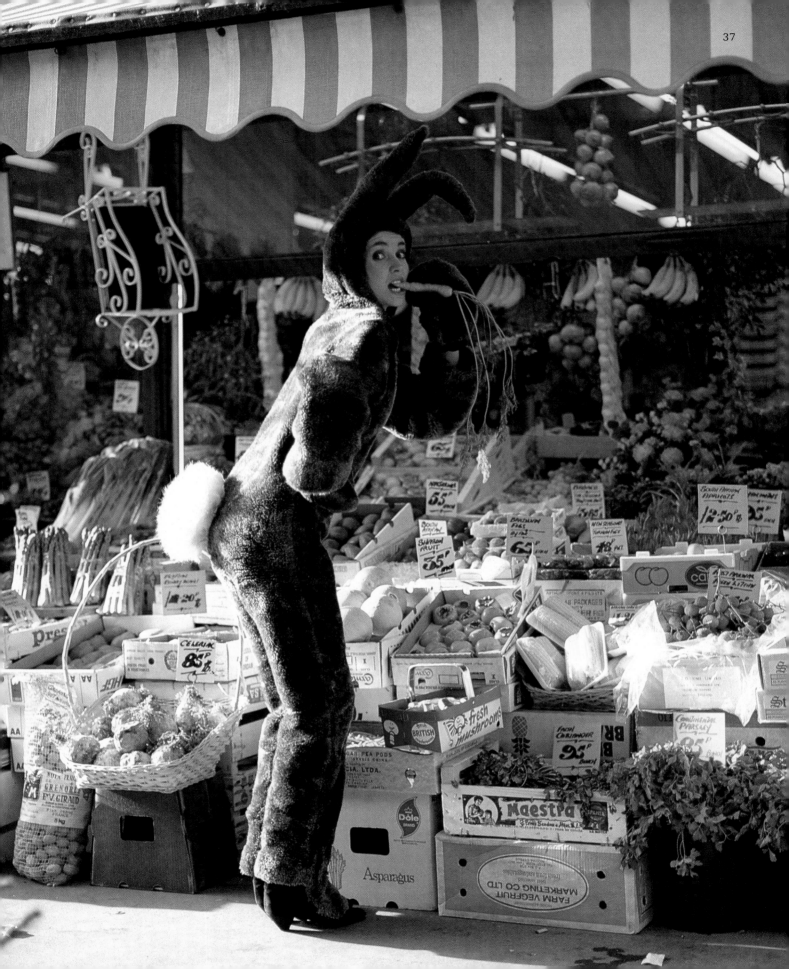

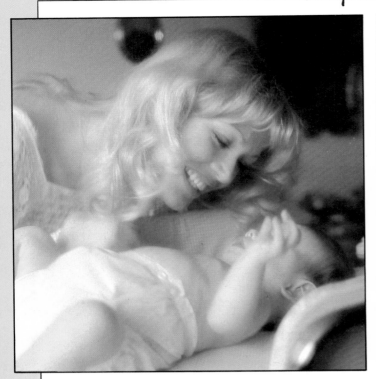

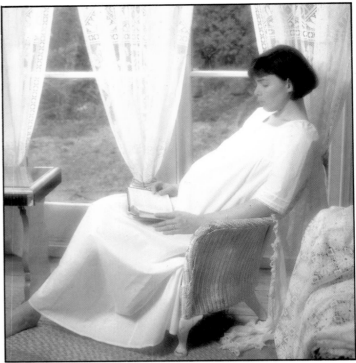

Start eating well before you are pregnant and you will be giving your child a better chance than if you start once you know you are: development starts very early. From then on, mother and child are getting the best chance to bloom – and for babies to learn healthy eating habits as natural.

Dad's eating habits matter too: children learn by example. Slim people shouldn't assume they eat healthily: quality is as important as the right quantity.

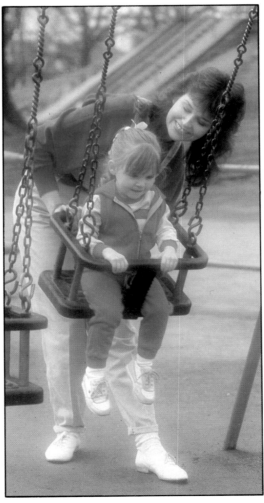

Many people think that if you're slim, you must be healthy, but look around you and you'll see that it isn't true. Some slim people don't eat much and may be undersupplied with nourishment; no wonder they don't sparkle with vitality. Others eat, but for one reason or another – physical or that stomach-churning tension – don't absorb food very efficiently or burn it off. It's just as important to look after your health by eating well if you're fashionably slender, as if you are struggling with your weight.

Most important of all is the way that mothers eat, both before and during pregnancy. Because the major development of a baby occurs very early in pregnancy, a woman changing to a healthy diet only when she discovers she's pregnant, some six or more weeks after conception, is far from ideal. It would be better if every woman planning a baby were to eat healthily for at least three months before conceiving.

Mothers and fathers of young children have another reason for healthy eating: children start copying what their parents do at a very early age. Why should a child avoid sweets if he sees Dad taking a bar of chocolate for his lunchbox, or Mum piling sugar into her tea?

The following five chapters offer guidelines that nutrition experts recommend.

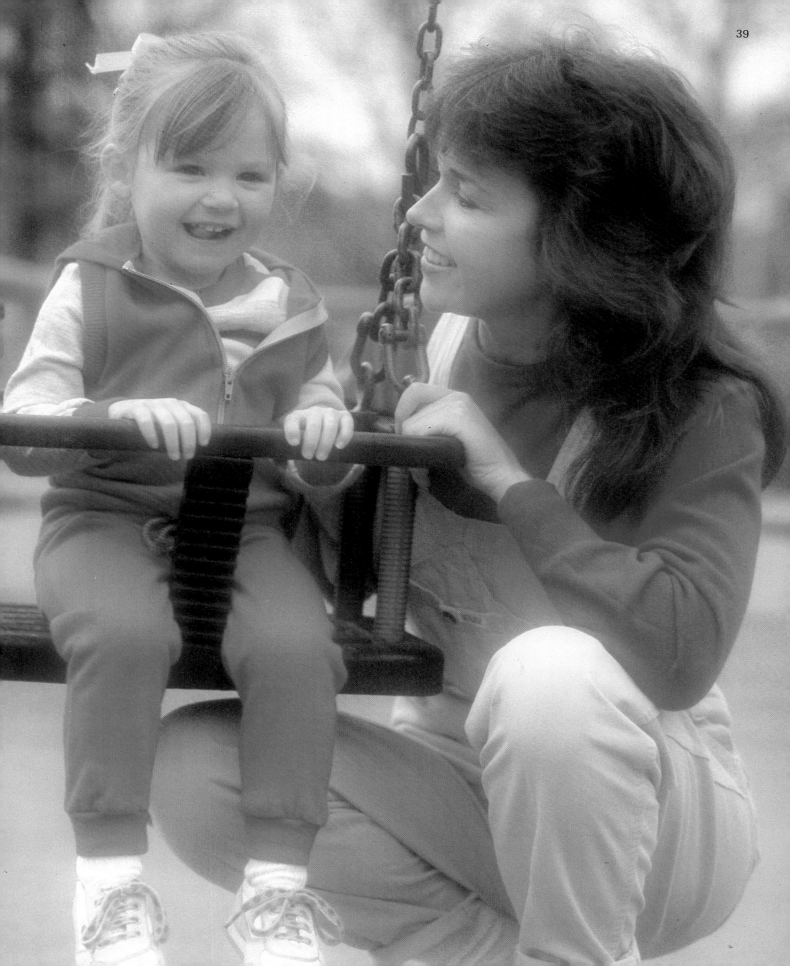

CHAPTER 3

Fats and a Healthy Diet

At the moment, the average Westerner gets around 4 out of every 10 calories he eats in the form of fat. That doesn't mean that 40% of what we eat is fat. Fat has twice as many calories as most other foods, so you only need to eat 20% of your food as fat to get that 40%. If someone eats around 2,000 calories a day, the 40% of calories can be produced by just over 88 grams, or 3 ounces, of fat a day. One gram of fat produces about 9 calories, so 88 grams is about 800 calories.

Provided we aren't overweight, why does the proportion of fat consumed matter? Because it's about twice as much fat as we need for good health and the extra can harm us. Too much fat doesn't only encourage overeating and overweight. Populations with a high fat diet have much higher rates of heart disease; and other health problems – such as the West's high incidence of gallstones – may be linked with excess fat.

There's suspicion that other 'epidemics of the 20th century' are at least partly linked with too much fat in our diet. They include the rising rate of diabetes, cancer of the breast and cancer of the colon or large intestine. Women used to be concerned about heart disease mainly on behalf of their men, and men are still much more prone to heart problems, but the rate is rising among younger women. Although eating too much fat is certainly not the sole cause – another may be more heavy smokers among women – it certainly doesn't help.

Why we are eating more fat? A major reason seems to be that we're better off. In the past, the main foods in the meals of almost everyone, except the wealthy few, were bread, potatoes, vegetables and beans. They're all very low in fat, but between them they provide enough protein for good health. With the advent of higher incomes and more food products, people were able to choose more of what used to be 'luxury' foods, like meat, dairy foods and eggs. By switching more of our food to these, we still get plenty of protein – more than we need in fact – but we unintentionally get a lot of fat, too. Even the leanest rump steak, for instance, has more than twice as much fat as bread; while beans and vegetables have hardly any.

At the same time, the kind of fat we eat has changed. Fats that are hard at room temperature – like most, but not all, animal fats – are known as saturated, because the bonds in their chemical structure are filled by hydrogen atoms and are hence incapable of undergoing additional reactions. It seems that these fats are more likely to raise the level of fat in the bloodstream. It's fats collecting in the bloodstream, gradually leaving deposits on the inside of artery walls, that eventually leads to the arteries becoming blocked or to clot formation, both being causes of heart attacks. If a clot lodges in the brain's arterial blood supply, restricting oxygenated flow, the result is a stroke. The story isn't a simple one, and fats certainly aren't the only cause – smoking, lack of exercise and reactions to stress are others – but hard fats are one factor we can change.

Fats which are liquid, but still thick, at room temperature, make up most of those which are called unsaturated; they could take a few more hydrogen atoms. From a health point of view, they seem to be neutral. Countries where such fats are the main ones used, such as olive oil in Greece, don't have particularly high rates of heart disease; in fact, much lower rates than the hard fat using communities.

Fats which are thoroughly runny at room temperature are called polyunsaturated, because their chemical structure has room for many more hydrogen atoms. These are the vegetable oils, such as sunflower, safflower, soya and corn. Others hover between polyunsaturated and unsaturated. These fats are not associated with a build-up of fats in arteries. On the other

Exercise won't undo bad eating habits, although it will help you eat plenty of food (increasing your chance of getting plenty of vitamins and minerals) – without getting fat. But you have to run a long, long way to work off calories if you don't change your diet as well.

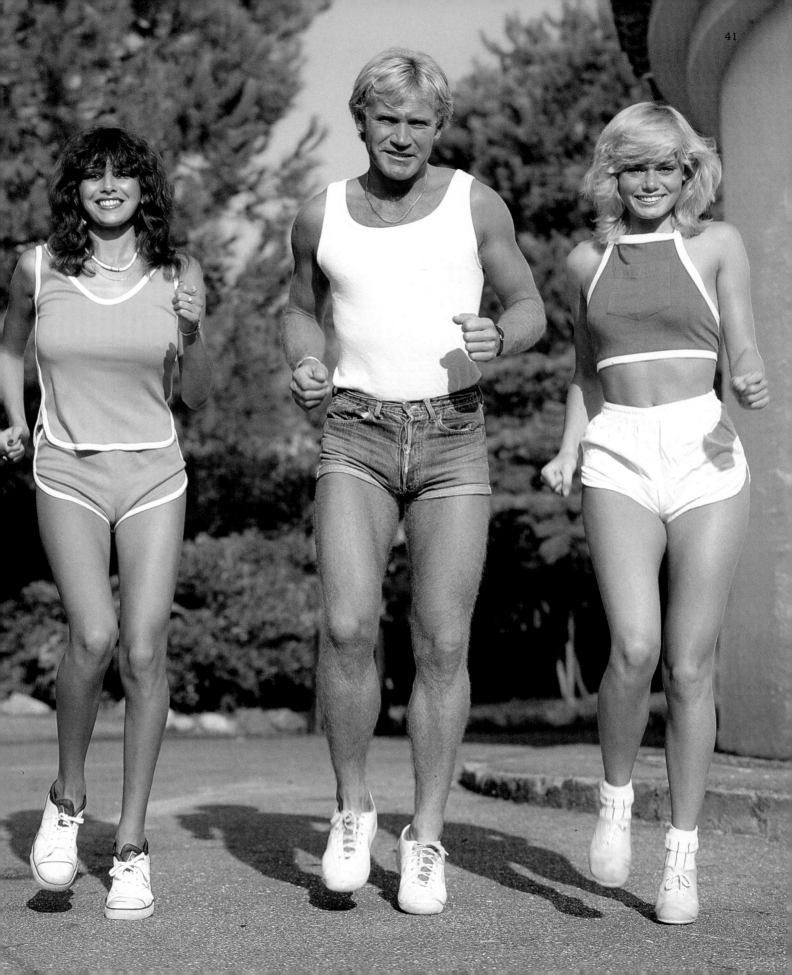

hand, they have just as many calories and overweight is, in itself, a contributor to many illnesses as far apart as aching joints and heart disease.

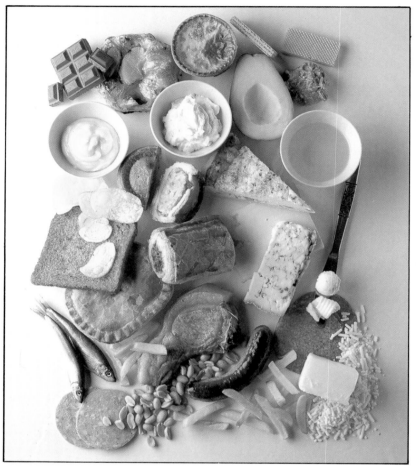

Above: high fat foods to be wary of, because you may not realise just how fatty they are – such as mayonnaise on salad (79% oil) or chocolate (30% fat). Don't say 'never', say 'hardly ever' – and tuck into the spread (opposite) of tasty, low fat foods, from trout to pasta. The bowls contain (from left): low fat soft cheese, ideal for making dips, dressings for salad, cheesecakes with less fat or instead of cream; low fat yoghurt; cultured buttermilk and smetana – like sour cream, but with less fat.

Fat is Important for Health Never aim for a fat-free diet. Fats are important for a whole range of body functions. Animal fats are the main sources of one form of vitamin A, retinol, and of vitamin D, which is necessary for the body to absorb calcium. We can get both vitamins from other sources. Another, but just as useful form of vitamin A, is the provitamin called carotene, which is rich in orange and yellow vegetables and fruit, and in leafy greens. The action of sunlight – it doesn't have to be shining – on the skin results in the formation of vitamin D. However, northern winters don't allow for much sunbathing and most people don't eat many vegetables.

The polyunsaturated fats provide important substances, which we don't get anywhere else, called 'essential fatty acids'. The body relies on food to provide them, instead of being able to make them, as it can some nutrients, from other ingredients in food.

The main item you need is called linoleic acid. It's rich in oils like safflower, sunflower (and in sunflower seeds), soya and corn. Linoleic acid is necessary for several body functions to work properly.

A popular way of getting linoleic acid is in soft margarine, but unless the packet is labelled 'high in polyunsaturates', don't bother; it may not be a good source. Some soft margarines now give the linoleic acid content on the label. It's usually got the words 'cis-cis' next to it. This mystifying term means that the linoleic acid hasn't been artificially hardened, which would spoil it. Have you ever wondered how margarine can be made from liquid oils? The answer is that some are hardened by a process called hydrogenation. As the name suggests, this involves making the polyunsaturated fat fill up its multiple bonds with hydrogen, which turns it into something hard like the saturated fats. Unfortunately, the artificially hardened fats end up different in structure from natural hard fats and they may be worse for our health, so avoid hard margarines. In the soft margarines labelled 'high in polyunsaturates', they've hardened just the minimum of oil to produce a solid-enough consistency, while keeping the high level of polyunsaturates or PUFAs. But while we all need some polyunsaturates, we only need an estimated 15 grams or ½ ounce a day at the most.

The aim is still to eat less fat of all kinds, although you are better off cutting the hard animal fats. Just to confuse things, not all hard fats are animal in origin. Palm and coconut 'oil', for example, are both solid and naturally saturated. Palm oil is often used in margarines. Animal fats which are soft, like fish oil, contain a high proportion of unsaturated and PUFAs, while semi-hard ones like chicken fat contain a mixture of saturated and unsaturated.

The aim is to eat only 2 spoonfuls of fat for every 3 you eat now.

Eating Less Fat You may think that you already eat little fat. Perhaps you're right, but most people are surprised to learn how much fat is 'hidden' in food. To eat less fat, go warily with all high fat foods, as well as the obvious steps of avoiding fried foods and spreading less margarine or butter on bread. It doesn't mean you must never eat them. Keep them for occasional, not everyday, use though even then the use of a little fat is fine.

Don't damn all high fat content foods as 'rubbish'. Some are full of food value, as well

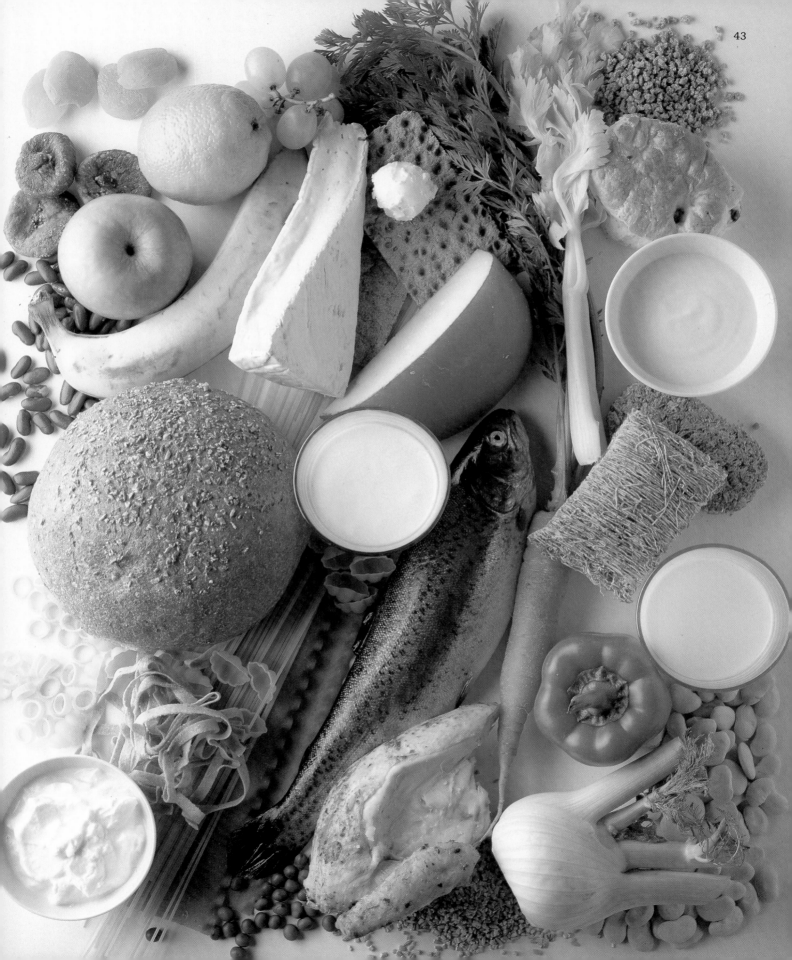

Fats and a Healthy Diet

Opposite: fats worth keeping because these foods contain other useful nutrients: eggs, nuts, oily fish like herring, a little safflower, sunflower or soya oil, and wheat germ – delicious added to cereals and puddings.
Oily fish like sardines and mackerel have a different kind of fat from most animal hard fats: their soft oil is more useful to the body, along with the vitamins A and D they're so rich in.

as the fat which means you shouldn't eat too much of them. The 'goodies' to keep in mind for occasional enjoyment are: peanuts and peanut butter, which are packed with protein, B vitamins and other goodness; avocado pears, containing vitamins A and E; herrings, a rich food for vitamins A and D, with mainly PUFA-type fats; and hard cheese for its high protein, vitamin B and calcium content.

On the other hand, some of the following foods have few redeeming features; keep them for a blue moon! They include fried bread, crisps, mayonnaise, chocolate, cream cheese, savoury and sweet pastries (pastry is always high in fat, especially when it is the puff or flaky type), pork chops and other fatty meats and pies, suet and most commercial biscuits.

There's still plenty left to eat; just look at our appetising low fat foods which can become the 'regulars' on your shopping list. Of course, without all that fat they are also very much lower in calories. So you either save calories and lose weight, or eat more of them and stay the same weight; you choose. You can also discover that eating less fatty foods won't make your meals more expensive.

How can you turn foods like pasta and beans into delicious meals without adding fat to them? Here are some secrets of low fat cooking:

1 When you're browning an onion or greasing a pan, use a new bristle paintbrush dipped in cooking oil, instead of pouring oil or adding a dollop of fat. You'll use far less fat and the recipe will work as well. Don't use a nylon bristled brush, or it will melt if it meets a hot pan.

2 Use fish and the least fatty meats. Even apparently lean meat has a surprising amount of fat hidden in it. The meat with the least hidden fat is turkey, followed by rabbit, chicken and then game, which also has more PUFAs and less saturated fats. White fish is leanest of all, followed by trout, salmon and then the oilier fish. But even oily fish, apart from eel and mackerel, is leaner than most meat.

3 Use more non-meat recipes. You may think that bread, rice and pasta are 'just stodge' but, in fact, they provide enough protein for main meals and contain almost no fat, as is the case with beans and lentils. Dishes like risotto, pizza, sandwiches and baked beans are all low in fat, provided you don't add too much. Be mean with oil when cooking, spreading bread or when adding cheese. Pick low fat sandwich fillings, such as chicken, low fat cheese, salad, yeast

extract, mashed bananas or apple slices. Sprinkle these last two with orange or lemon juice so they don't go brown.

4 Remember that most of us eat much more protein than we need. So use more light salad meals and plain bread or potatoes to replace the fancier, rich foods.

Useful Fats Here are some foods which have a high level of fat, but which also contain so much goodness that it's a good idea to keep them on your shopping list; just use them a little less often than normal. Because their fats are still in the food and unprocessed, they are fresher and more natural.

✳ Use 3-4 eggs a week – the national average – if you like them.

✳ Herrings provide the richest source of vitamins A and D, plus useful minerals, B vitamins and vitamin E. In winter, when vitamin D from the action of sunlight on skin is in short supply, it's a good idea to eat oily fish once a week.

✳ Nuts provide protein, B vitamins and vitamin E, plus useful minerals. They also contain plenty of fibre. Use small helpings to add flavour and protein to vegetable and rice dishes, but not more than 40 to 55 grams (1½-2oz) per person for a main dish. Hazelnuts are much less fatty than the others; walnuts highest in PUFA, although they all contain some; almonds and sunflower seeds are good for protein, along with peanuts.

✳ Wheat germ is so packed with protein (25% – more than meat), B group vitamins and vitamin E, it's as good as a vitamin pill! Sprinkle a tablespoonful here and there on cereals, stewed fruit or savouries, but after cooking so the goodness won't get cooked out of it. Wheat germ goes stale quickly, so keep it in the refrigerator and use it within a few weeks while it's still sweet in flavour. Throw it away if it goes bitter.

✳ Oils are the most natural way, apart from nuts and seeds, to get the vital PUFAs. Keep sunflower, safflower and soya oil for use on salads. They burn too easily to be heated to high temperatures, but are fine in baking. For frying, olive and corn oil are the most stable. In health food stores, you'll see 'cold-pressed oils' for sale. These are thicker and have more flavour. They are extracted from the plant by pressure, rather than by heat or chemical treatment. They're expensive, but they are more natural. As you are aiming for a low fat diet, you won't use much, so why not buy the best?

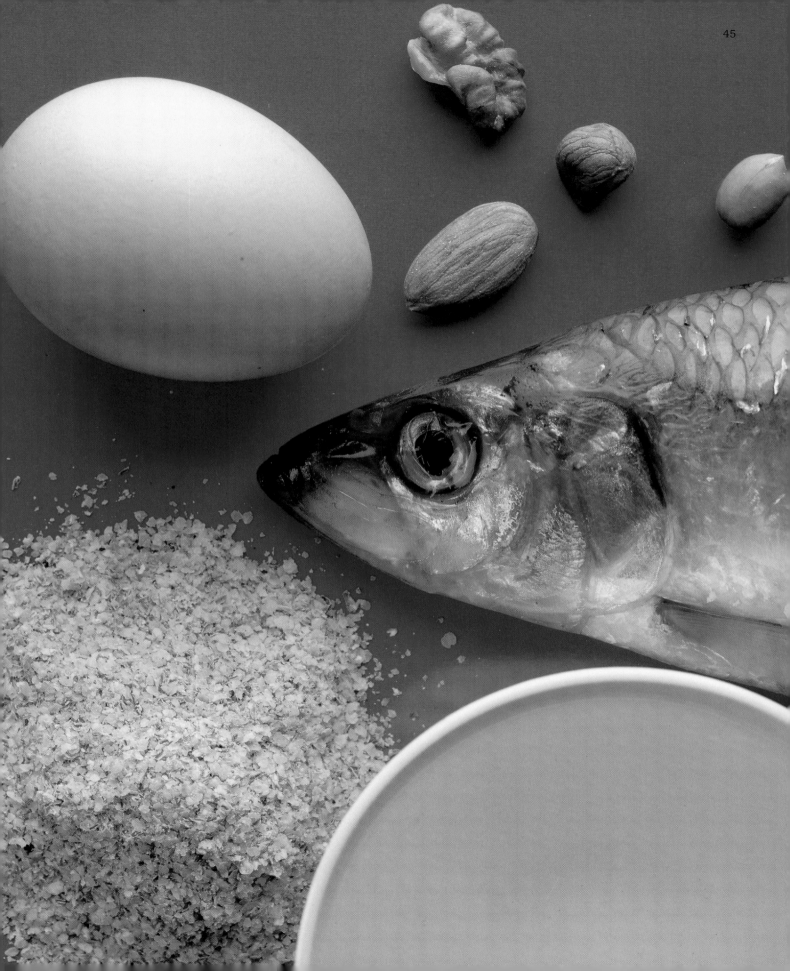

46

CHAPTER 4

Sugar and a Healthy Diet

Sugar is so more-ish, it's the main feature of 'bingeing'. It's often done for comfort, but leads to the opposite – self-hate. The urge can be transferred to harmless, more filling foods like bananas. Because they are very low in fat, you'll find it hard to tuck away too many calories – you'll get too full.

Everyone knows that sugar is bad for your teeth, but what other reasons are there for saying we should eat less of it? The main argument is that sugar contains no vitamins, minerals or other substances useful and necessary for health. So eating sugar, while it supplies calories or energy, is pushing out of our meals other foods which would provide important nutrients.

Because sugar is so concentrated, it's easy to eat too much of it, and anyone who has ever 'eaten for comfort' will recognise that eating sugar is sometimes almost irresistible. When people go on a food 'binge', it's almost always sugary foods – from chocolate to doughnuts – that they crave. You'd be surprised how many people have eaten their way through half a dozen or more such items, one after the other, when upset about something.

The old phrase 'You are what you eat' has never seemed truer than when you're looking at a cream bun fan, who often looks as though the cream is just about to squidge out of her rounded frame! Why say 'her'? Although some men also crave sweet foods, the unconscious use of sweet and sticky foods as an outlet for emotion when upset seems mainly to affect women. Men seem more likely to turn to alcohol or other outlets.

It's important not to get the idea that cream cakes are somehow 'wicked'. That may just make them seem more desirable, or make you feel horribly guilty when you eat one. Eating the occasional cake, bar of chocolate, gateau or pastry never hurt anyone. It shouldn't be a reason for feeling a failure, even if you're trying to lose weight. Just enjoy it and then go back to eating healthily. Don't go the other way and feel so bad – 'I've ruined my diet' – that you promptly eat a plateful more of sweet stodge.

If you know you are one of those people who can't open a bar or box of chocolates without wolfing the lot, it's safest to keep

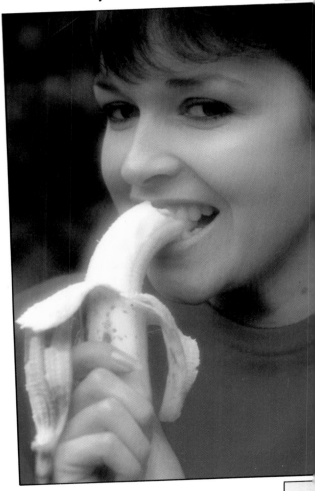

away from sugar almost all the time. However, if you can cope, a little sugar – say up to 25g (1oz) per day – is unlikely to harm you. It won't do you any good either, but it's a lot less than most people eat. The national average is a colossal 110g (3⅞oz) approximately each day from food and drink, including alcohol. That means that some women are eating their weight in sugar each year, and many more of us are almost achieving this dubious feat. No wonder official reports would like us to eat less sugar and replace it with other foods

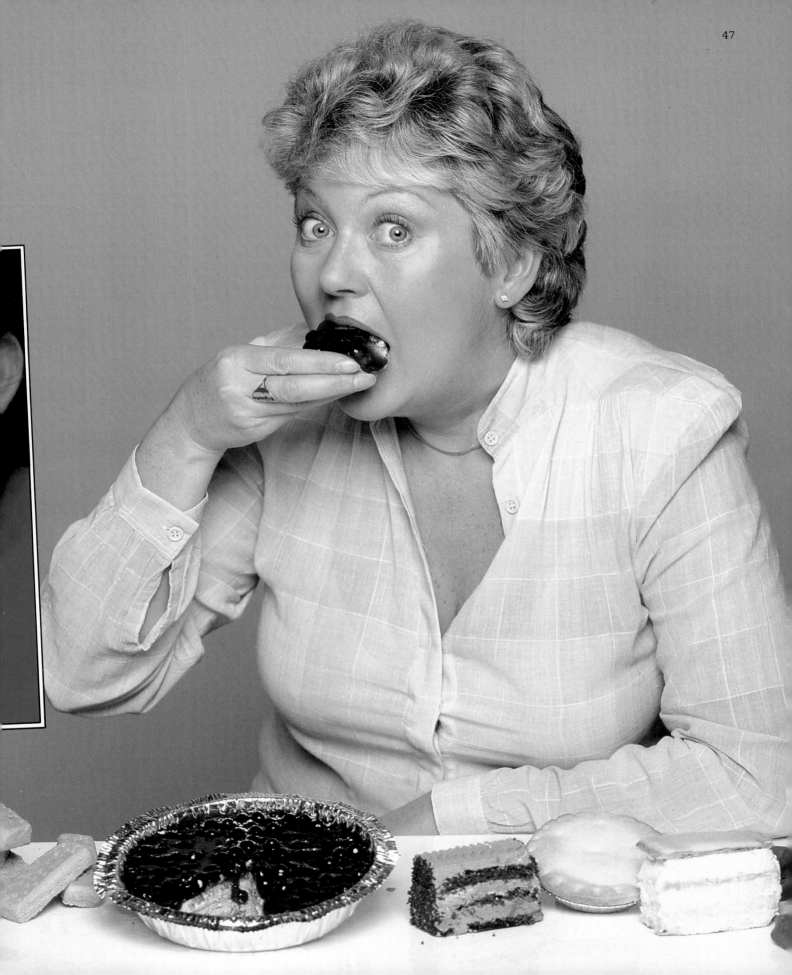

which provide something more useful to the body.

Don't we need sugar for energy? Sugar does provide energy, which is just another word for calories, but so do many other foods. Sugar doesn't have any magical, special energy. Your body can turn almost anything you eat into energy.

sugar. While we all know that buns and cakes contain sugar, some contain very much more than others. With some foods, reading the label is a guide to how much sugar has been added. Ingredients are listed in descending order of weight. So a food product with an ingredients list showing sugar at, or near the top, means

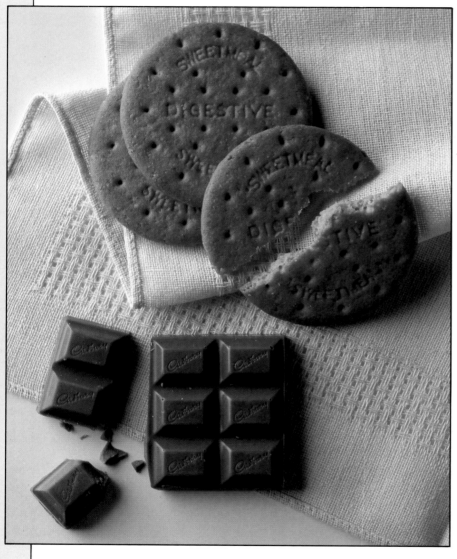

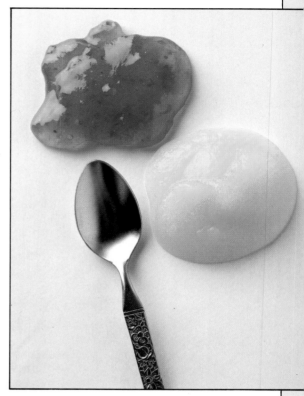

that it has a higher proportion of sugar than a similar product with sugar near the bottom of the list. This is a useful point to remember when deciding which kind of breakfast cereal, pickle or biscuit to buy.

Here are eight pairs of foods, all sweet. However, one of each pair has considerably more sugar than the other.

Currant bun, average 14% sugar.
Blackcurrant cream tartlet; fancy cakes average 54% sugar.

Digestive biscuits, average 16% sugar.
Milk chocolate – ½ a 100-gram bar – average 56% sugar.

Dry wine, average 0.6% sugar.
Sweet wine, average 6% sugar.

Tomato ketchup, average 23% sugar.
Marmalade, average 70% sugar.

Black cherry yogurt, average 14% sugar, or 20g (¾oz) per 5oz pot.
Plain yogurt with grapes, average 13%

The invisible difference: three examples of why it pays to get to know where invisible sugar in food is – so you can dodge it and enjoy the less-sweet alternative.

Eating Less Sugar As your body doesn't need crystal sugar at all, you can trim as much as you want from your meals without any fear of ill-effects. It's easiest to trim the sugar you can see: any you add to drinks, cereal or puddings, and also any sweets you eat, or sweet drinks.

These are the most obvious sugars to reduce, but one reason why we eat so much sugar is that sugar is an invisible ingredient in many common foods. Do you think of jam as mainly fruit or mainly sugar, for instance? By law, it can be two-thirds

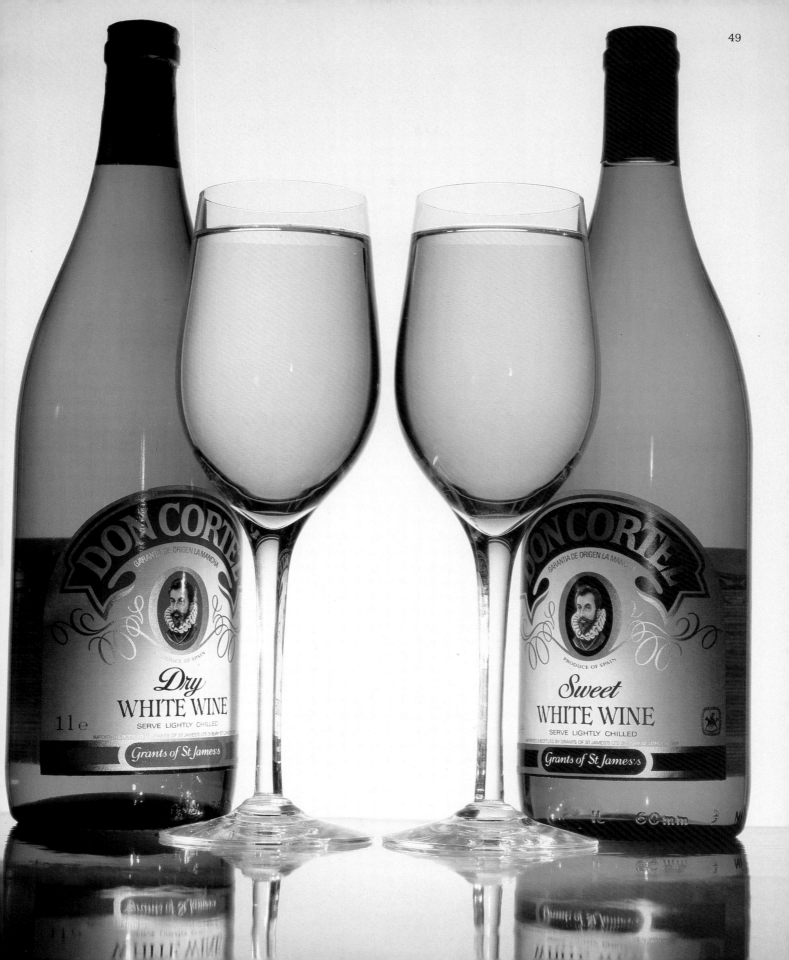

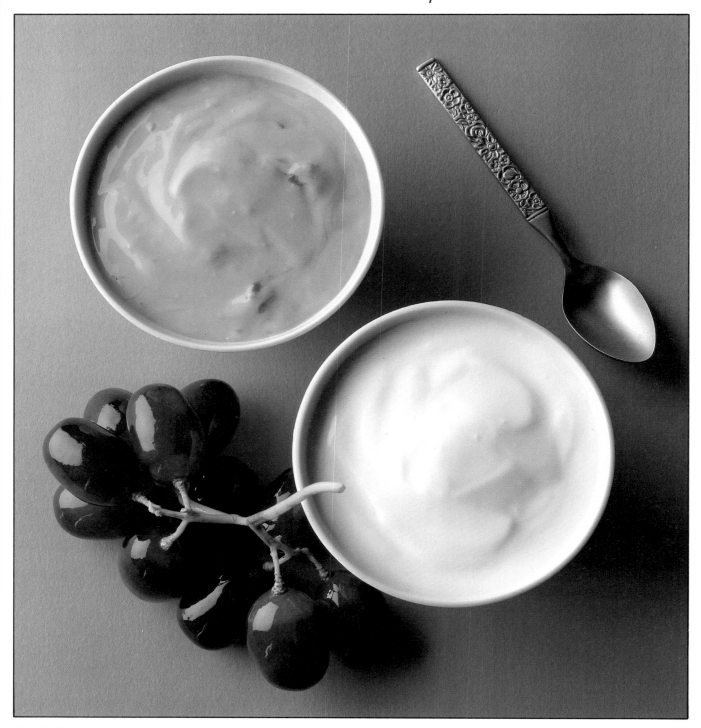

More 'hidden' sugars: there's always something nice to eat that has less sugar. Your tastebuds will quickly adapt too, so that you find high sugar foods too sweet.

natural sugars, but to eat 20g (¾oz), you can eat 10½oz fruit and yogurt.

Strawberry jam, average 69% sugar.
Apple purée with the minimum of honey or sugar, average 10% sugar.

Cornflakes with 2 tsp sugar, average 7% and 100% sugar respectively, giving about ½oz sugar per helping of 1oz cornflakes with sugar.

Porridge with 2 tsp bran, average sugar negligible.

Apricot chutney, average 50% sugar.
Piccalilli pickle, average 2.6% sugar.

So, you can often choose a replacement for a very sweet food that does the job, or satisfies your sweet tooth, but has only a fraction of the sugar. The sugar in fruit and milk, by the way, can almost be discounted

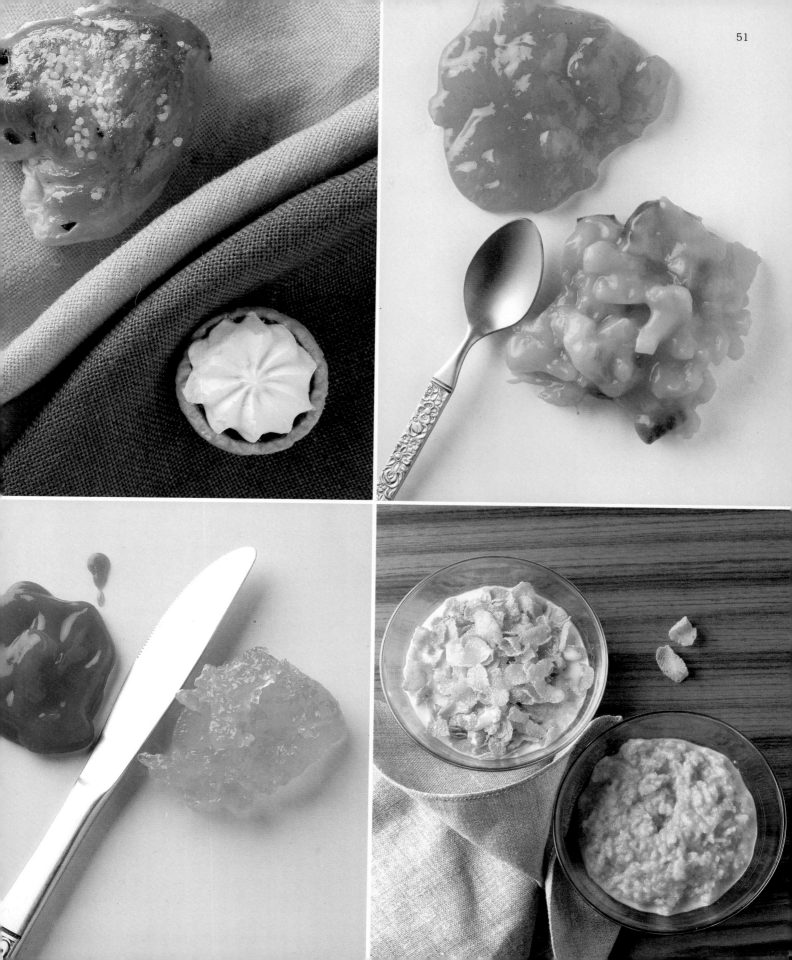

because it's well diluted, so you don't get such a large amount, and it's treated differently by your digestive system.

Is there anything you can sweeten food with that's better for you than sugar is?

Here's a guide to alternative sweeteners. Some are much better than sugar, but it has to be said that the healthiest move is to eat less sweet things in general. Your taste buds will adapt and you'll find you aren't tempted by sweets and cakes nearly so much. If you do ever slip back to sweet foods, you may find that they taste revoltingly sickly!

Below: starting with the dark honey at the top, go anti-clockwise for molasses sugar, Demerara sugar, fruit sugar, aspartame (artificial sweetener), saccharin, and muscovado sugar – see page 54 for details.

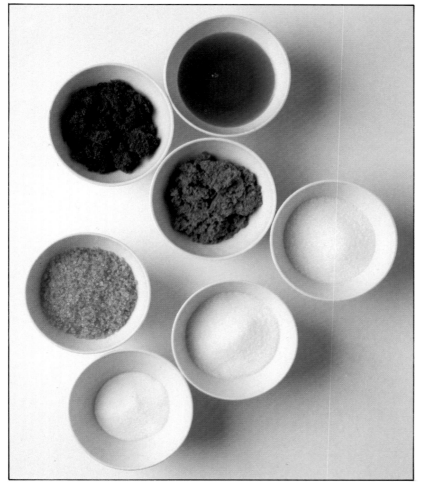

Opposite: anti-clockwise from top: molasses, black treacle, sultanas, maple syrup, concentrated apple juice, dates and dried apricots – the natural sweeteners with advantages over sugar in more refined, crystal form.

Molasses: thick, almost black syrup left when sugar cane is boiled and the sugar extracted. Contains only about half as much sugar and has such a strong flavour, you'd find it impossible to eat a lot. However, useful for adding a taste-plus-sweetness to gingerbread, milk drinks, stewed fruit or porridge. It also has roughly only half the calories of sugar, plus useful minerals, especially iron, calcium and magnesium. Fine if you only use say 2

tablespoons a day, otherwise its laxative properties will begin to take effect.

Black treacle: taken from another stage in the refining process, it has a little more sugar and calories, rather less but still useful amounts of minerals, and makes a less dramatic impact with its flavour. Fine in small amounts, it has a laxative effect, like molasses, if you take more than a spoonful or two.

Sultanas: together with raisins, these are one of the best sweeteners. At around 71 calories per 28 grams (1oz), they are still very sweet, but 'pay' for their calories with fibre, minerals and a small amount of B vitamins. Use them in small amounts instead of sweets (but remember that you should still clean your teeth afterwards), and in cooking. The way to get most sweetness from them is to liquidise washed sultanas or raisins with the liquid in a recipe before cooking. If you like sweet cereal, for instance, liquidise the fruit in the milk you are going to pour over it. You can use the same technique to sweeten stewed fruit, doing the blending before adding the sweetened water to the raw fruit and cooking.

Maple syrup: is more like honey in composition than sugar, so see the reference to honey for ideas on its use. Make sure that what you buy is genuine maple syrup and not maple flavour syrup, which will be just flavoured sugar syrup. The real thing is expensive but has a delicious flavour, which should help you enjoy even small amounts.

Concentrated apple juice: is mainly used as an economical way of making apple drinks; you just add hot or cold water. It's certainly better for you than soft drinks high in sugar, colourings and often caffeine. It's still sweet, without the addition of sugar. You can also use it to sweeten dishes, too, provided you keep to small amounts because it is quite acidic under the sweetness. Good uses include in fruit cakes, or when you want a touch of sweetness in a curry or casserole; a tablespoon goes quite a long way. To make an apple drink, just use like a concentrated fruit drink.

Dates: are the most useful natural sweetener for making fruit cakes and puddings. They're very sweet indeed. A good way to use them is to prepare a purée by cooking dates in enough water to cover, until you have a soft consistency. Make sure the mixture contains no stones, then purée

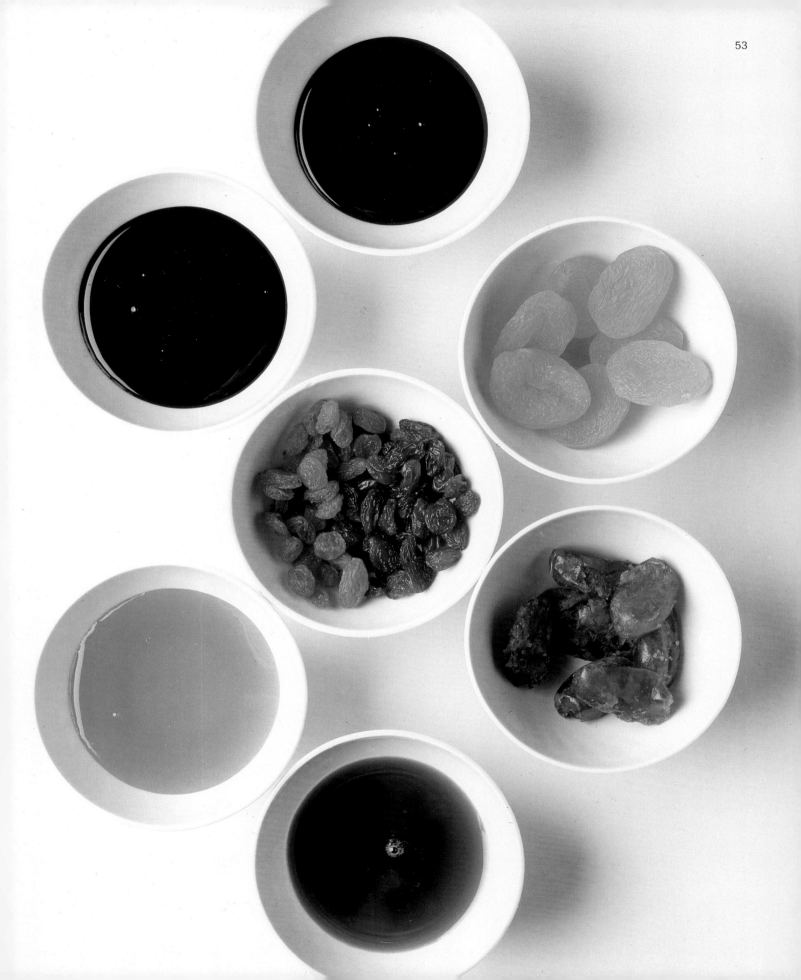

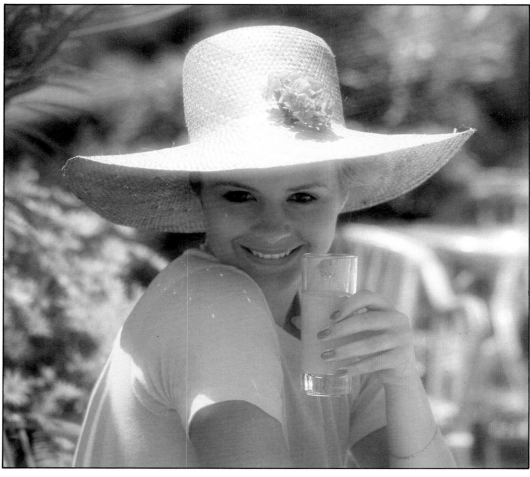

Right: unsweetened fruit juice is sweet enough for most of us, so why add ounces of sugar to other foods and drinks?
Opposite: no, you don't need to eat sugar 'for energy'. You can swim, run or play sports just as energetically on any other food. The body can turn all your meals into energy, and any food will give you more vitamins, minerals or fibre than sugar will.

in a blender or by mashing thoroughly with a fork. Use this purée, weight for weight, in place of the sugar required by the recipe, remembering to reduce the amount of liquid to allow for the extra water you've added. The easiest way to do this is to add liquid to the recipe cautiously until you've achieved the consistency the recipe suggests, which is much easier than measuring. This mixture contains about 70 calories per ounce.

Dried apricots: a versatile alternative to sugar as a source of sweetness, dried apricots can be munched as they are instead of sweets; stewed with sour fruit or porridge, which the apricots will sweeten; made into a thick purée, which can be used instead of jam to spread on bread, or to fill cake; or served stewed, hot or cold, as a sweet but nourishing pudding. They contain approximately 52 calories per ounce, under half the level in sugar, because their sweetness is diluted with a high level of fibre, as well as having one of the highest levels of vitamin A (in carotene form), iron and other useful nutrients. Before cooking or eating apricots it's useful,

if possible, to boil them in some water, simmer for a minute or two, then drain, throwing the water away. This is an effective way of cleaning them and also helps to remove some of the preservative sulphur dioxide which keeps them pale. It is sometimes possible to buy darker 'unsulphured' apricots.

Honey: is sometimes treated by nutritionists as no better than sugar, but it does have advantages. These are, first, that it contains fewer calories: roughly 82 per ounce, versus sugar's 110. Second, it is somewhat sweeter, especially when added to cold foods, so you may use less. Third, a major part of its sweetness is in a form which is more slowly released to the body as energy, a useful property for diabetics or those with diabetic tendencies who need to avoid sudden surges in the level of energy supplied to the body. On the other hand, don't replace a high level of sugar with a high intake of honey and expect to gain greatly. Honey contains small amounts of many minerals and vitamins, but such small amounts that it contributes only tiny quantities compared

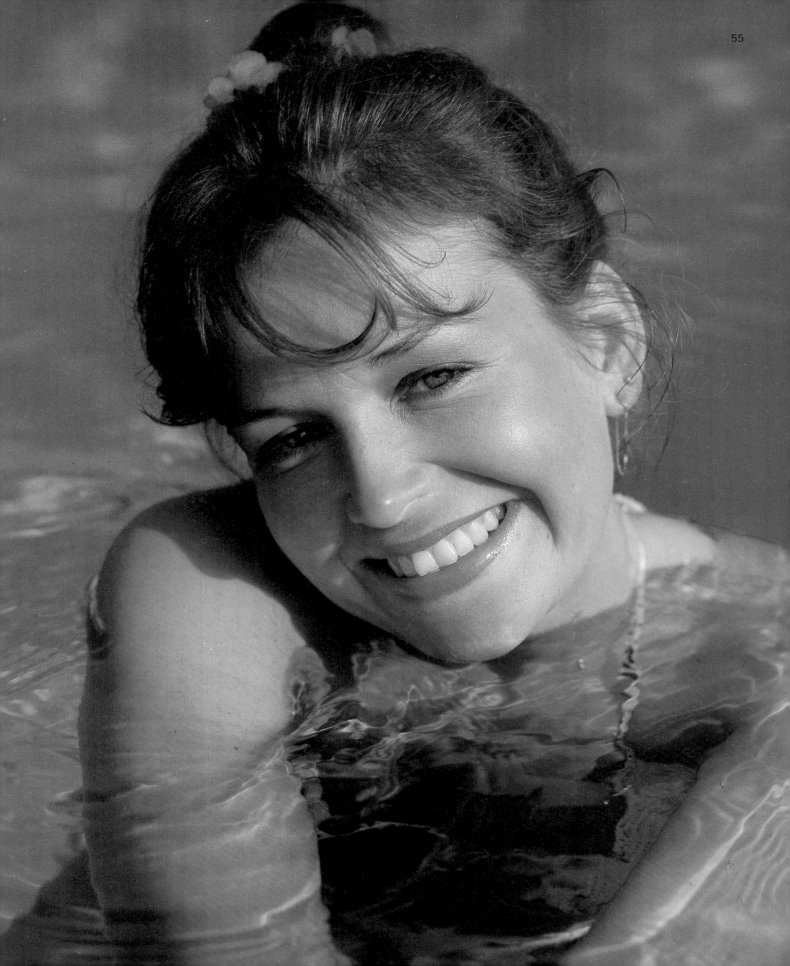

Opposite: snacks to remember next time you get that craving for something sweet. From an apple sandwich to a health food shop no-added-sugar fruit bar to a bowl of porridge with a little honey, you get more goodness for your calories, and usually fewer calories, this way.

to our needs. So it's wisest to treat it as a not particularly nutritious food, to be used to avoid the problems of sugar, but not in large quantities; one ounce a day, which is about one tablespoonful, would be sensible.

Molasses sugar: the most nourishing kind of sugar, molasses sugar has a strong, treacly taste but doesn't have a lot of vitamins and minerals. Use it sparingly; it's less worthwhile than molasses or black treacle and can overpower other ingredients with its strong flavour, if you use more than a spoonful or two. Like other sugars, it contains about 110 calories per ounce.

Demerara sugar: a few traces of minerals are all that make this sugar better than white. However, it is still that bit better, provided you don't use more than about one ounce per day. Another reason is that it has a flavour, unlike white sugar which is just sweet. This can make it a more effective flavouring agent in small amounts. Of brown sugars, this is the most versatile in cooking and for serving to guests to put in drinks; even though it's also the palest and one of the lowest in minerals. Contains 110 calories per ounce.

Fruit sugar: looks just like a fine-crystal white sugar, but once you taste it, it behaves differently. Firstly, it's considerably sweeter to most people's taste buds than sugar, especially when used in cold foods and drinks. This means that less need be used. Secondly, it provides a kind of sugar which is absorbed more slowly by the body as energy, which is good for diabetics – who should ask their medical advisor before using it – but also for those who react to sugar with a brief burst of energy, followed by a slump! Fruit sugar, also known as fructose or levulose, is extracted from plants and attracts water, so it needs to be stored in a tightly sealed jar. You can use it to replace sugar in many dishes, but use less both for the nutritional advantage and also

because it will produce more sweetness. You can't simply swop fruit sugar for ordinary sugar in baking sponges or jam-making; write to the manufacturer for special recipes. Fruit sugar is not particularly slimming, unless you use less than ordinary sugar; both contain 110 calories per ounce.

Aspartame: is the newest artificial sweetener. It's made from two proteins, so although it isn't natural, its 'parents' are. It contains almost no calories, so can be used just like saccharin, i.e. where sweetness is wanted, without the recipe requiring bulk. It contains phenylalanine, a natural amino acid which some people cannot tolerate, but this is labelled on the product and most people with this problem are well aware of it. Products based on aspartame are claimed not to have the bitter aftertaste associated with other artificial sweeteners.

Saccharin: is the longest-established and most widely used artificial sweetener. Doubts have been raised about its safety, but it is not proven that it has any ill-effects. You may prefer to avoid it for another reason: it certainly isn't natural and does not help you retrain your taste buds to want less sweetness. It contains no calories.

Muscovado sugar: available in dark and light versions, is the 'halfway house' between molasses sugar and demerara sugar, in both strength of flavour and in mineral content. Again, use it if you like it, but in small amounts, say around one ounce per day. It contains 110 calories per ounce.

What to eat when you get that craving for something sweet.
Here is a list of foods that give you sweetness and food value:

bowl of porridge with one tsp honey
oatcake, scone, banana
fruit bar, dried apricots, apple
wholemeal apple sandwich
wholemeal biscuit

Lifestyle Quiz

Quiz – Are You a Sugar Addict? Find out if you're an unconscious sugar 'addict' by answering these questions – truthfully!

1 *Is a day without something sweet unthinkable?* A. Yes. B. No.
2 *Do you find it hard to eat only part of a bar*
of chocolate or packet of chocolate biscuits?
A. Yes. B. No.
3 *Do you find you want sweet foods more when you're upset or bored?* A. Yes. B. No.
4 *Are you almost afraid to buy sweet foods, because you think you may wolf the lot?* A. Yes. B. No.

If you score more than two 'Yesses', you're fairly hooked, but don't give up hope. Once you realise how much you depend on sugar, it's easier to divert that attention

to another harmless, or even healthy activity, such as eating apples, gardening or cleaning your shoes when you get that sugary urge.

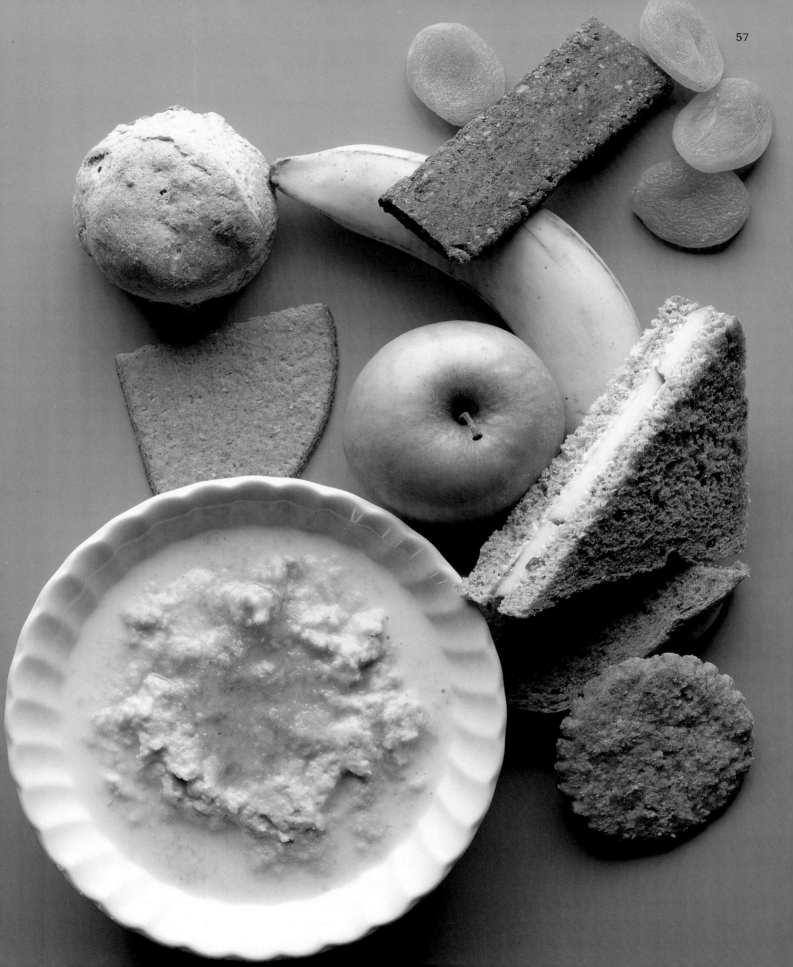

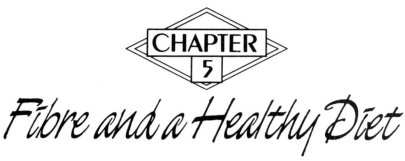

CHAPTER 5

Fibre and a Healthy Diet

As incomes have risen, Westerners have eaten less bread, rice, pasta, potatoes and all the other basic grains and carbohydrate foods. People have generally thought of this as 'progress'. The animal and dairy foods they eat instead contain more protein, they point out. For a long time, people also had the idea that these animal foods were less fattening, while thinking of bread and potatoes as 'just stodge'. Now expert opinion agrees that the change has not been a healthy one. It's had two main results: the foods we eat more of do have more protein, but they also have much more fat, and the foods we eat less of provided us with something very important that is now deficient in our diet – fibre.

Fibre is a 'family' word used to describe several substances found in the walls of plant cells. They all share the property that little of them is digested, so they pass through the body in roughly the same bulk in which they're eaten. This bulk 'pads out' the waste products of other foods eaten, so that the result is a neat and fairly large parcel that the muscles of the wall of the intestine can get a good grip on and move faster down the tube!

Comparisons between Westerners and natives of communities which still eat a lot of fibre, show that the latter are freer from several of the intestinal ailments which are virtual epidemics here. That doesn't prove the connection but this evidence, coupled with tests on the result of fibre in food here, are fairly convincing.

Eating more fibre is the easiest and most efficient way of avoiding or curing constipation, and also of making food travel more quickly through the body. This may have an advantage, some experts say, by shortening the time for which harmful waste products in food are in contact with the vulnerable, absorbent wall of the bowel. Other intestinal problems have been relieved by taking extra fibre – from

haemorrhoids to a common problem in older people, diverticulitis.

The message now is: eat more fibre foods. They are not so high in protein, but still high enough, since most of us eat very much more protein than we need. They are certainly no more fattening than most protein foods, since most meat, cheese and milk/cream products gain many extra calories from their high fat content. The exceptions are the lean meats, especially poultry, game, rabbit and turkey, and white fish, low fat cottage cheese and low fat yogurt. If you combine foods from this last list with fibre foods like bread, breakfast cereals and potatoes – but go easy on other, fattier animal foods – you can enjoy a surprising amount of the breads and pasta most of us enjoy and gain no weight, but have a better-balanced style of eating.

However, at the same time as the move from bread to beef was beginning, refining of flour changed to remove almost all the fibre from bread. It also removed most of the B vitamins and minerals, and some of the protein. White bread contains very little fibre; wholemeal or wholewheat bread (the same thing), about 3 times as much. It's the same story with pasta, rice and breakfast cereals. To get the fibre, and more vitamins and minerals, you need to choose the 'whole' version. These are once more widely available, as more and more people want to put the fibre back into what they eat. Also having a revival are the beans and lentils, which provide protein and fibre with very little fat. Fruit and vegetables, and nuts, are the third source of fibre. So eating more fruit and vegetables helps your health in more ways than one.

Because the fibres from different kinds of food behave differently inside us, it's wise to include all kinds of fibre in what we eat. Since it makes food bulkier, it can often mean that people feel fuller quickly and eat less. This is why changing to a high fibre style of eating can help people lose weight.

Opposite: feeling fresh comes from inside as well as out. Fibre helps your digestive system work briskly so waste products don't linger inside, slowing both you and your circulation.

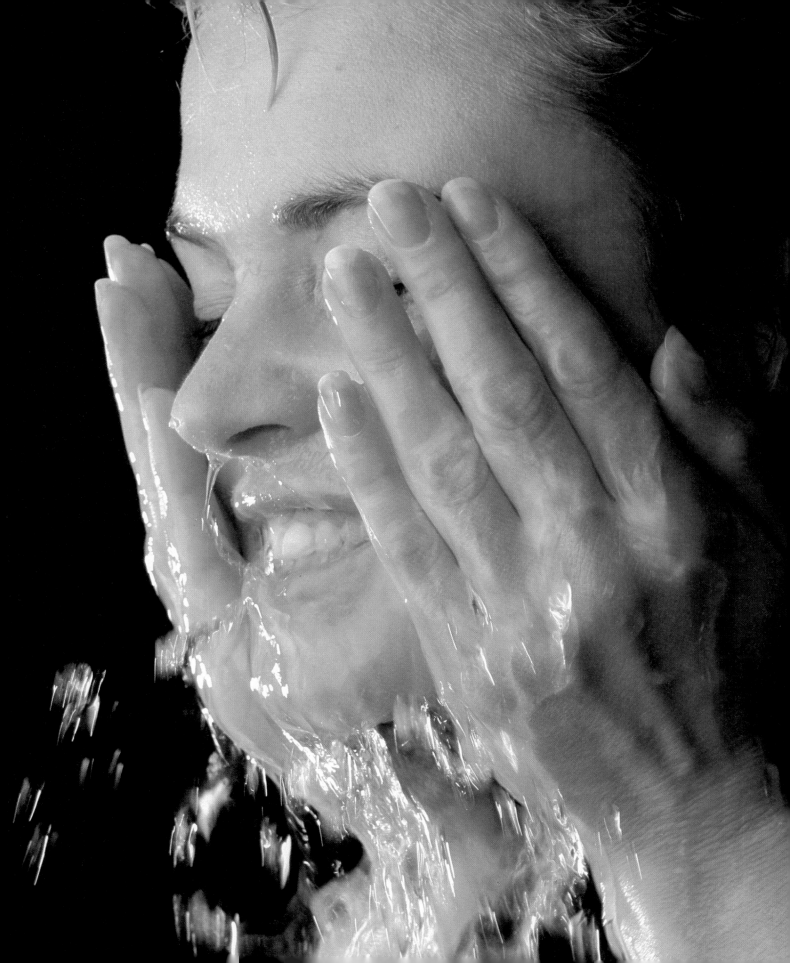

Eating More Fibre You'll eat more fibre automatically if you choose natural foods, rather than packaged, processed ones; and if you replace some of the animal foods you eat, such as cheese, eggs or meat, with vegetable protein foods, like grains or cereals, beans or lentils, fruit, nuts and vegetables. If you do this, and choose the wholemeal versions of rice, bread and so on, you won't need to add bran to food. It'll be built in to the foods you are eating.

Don't suddenly start stuffing yourself with high-fibre foods. If your digestive system isn't used to them, you're likely to react to large amounts by feeling 'blown out' and uncomfortable, because of the unaccustomed bulk. It's better to change over to more fibre foods over several weeks, or even a few months.

Aim regularly to include in your meals some from each of the following groups:

1 Wholemeal bread, pasta, or cereals, or wholemeal crispbread. Brown rice.

2 Oatmeal, porridge oats or oatcakes. Beans or lentils, in soups, stews, salads, dhal etc. Peas or broad beans.

3 Fruit and vegetables, especially soft fruit such as blackcurrants and leafy vegetables such as spinach; or runner beans; or sweet corn.

Right: don't think that eating fibre foods will make you feel bulky or give you a big tummy. On the contrary, they can help you stay slender.
Opposite: fibre isn't all bran. All these foods are especially rich in fibre – so put them on your shopping list. Clockwise from coconut: black-berries, sweetcorn, puffed cereals, prunes, runner beans, dried apricots, blackcurrants (and other soft fruit like raspberries), lentils, soya beans, brown rice, nuts of all kinds, passionfruit.

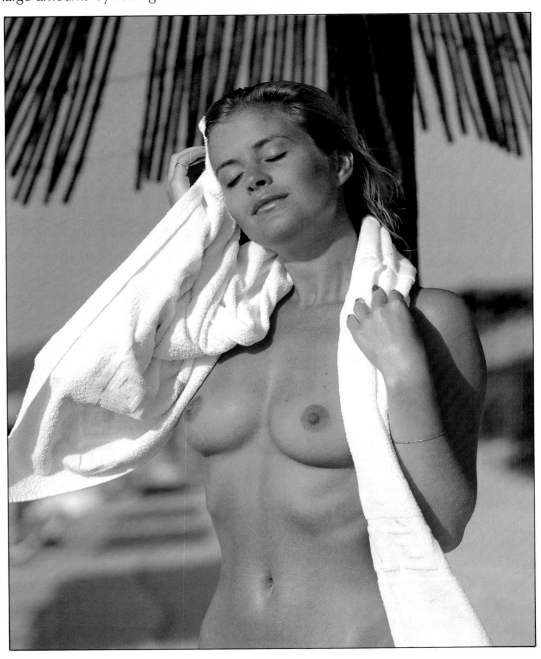

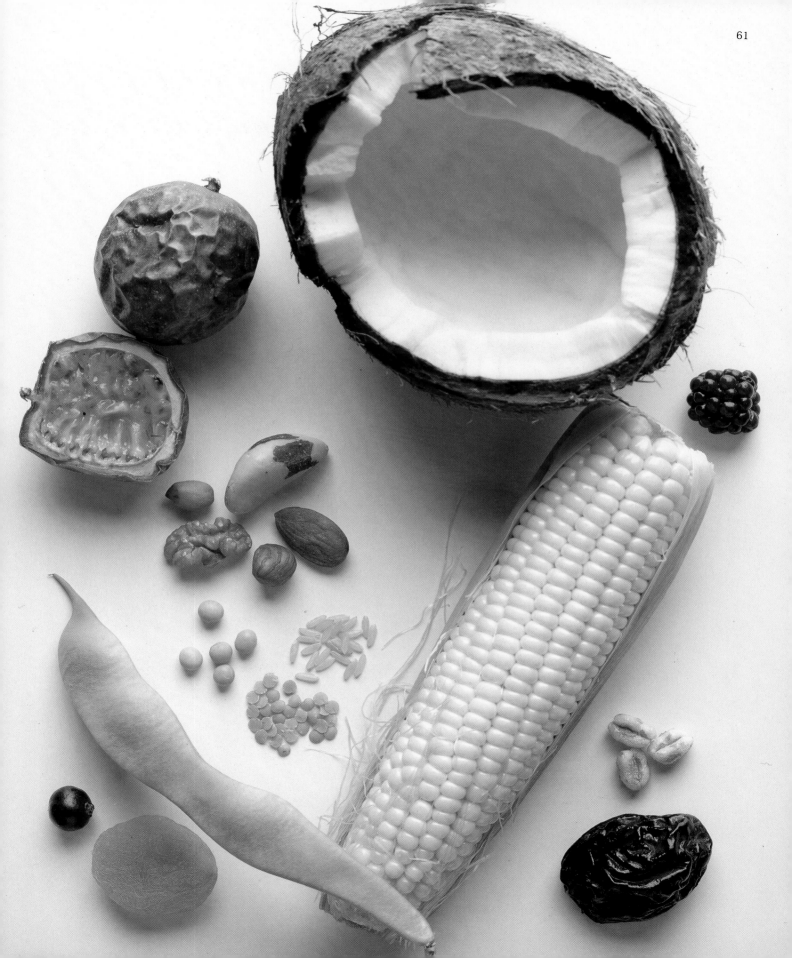

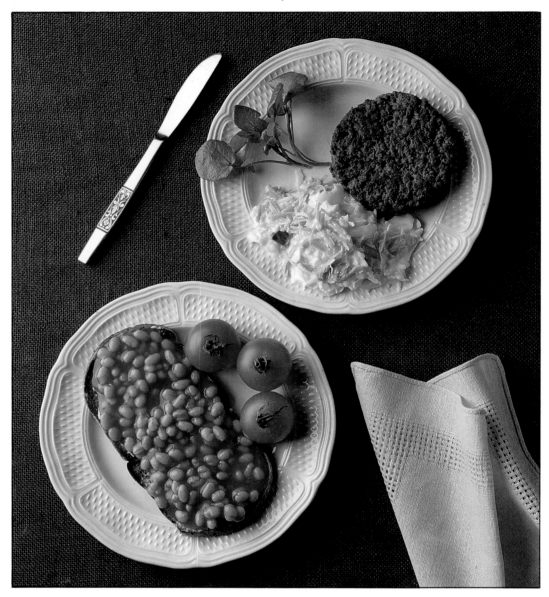

More carbohydrate can mean less calories. Right: grilled hamburger and coleslaw loses to less fatty, higher fibre baked beans on toast with tomatoes. Opposite: 'slimmer's' meal of steak and salad has more fat, and more calories than the egg salad sandwiches.

Here are examples of how meals with plenty of carbohydrate are healthier than the conventional equivalents:

1 *A 5oz beef hamburger with shop-bought coleslaw, versus 7oz baked beans on a slice of wholemeal toast, with 3 tomatoes.*

When you want a take-away meal, both these will generally be available. Choose the hamburger and you're clocking up about 16% fat, according to a Consumers' Association survey of minced beef; roughly 350 calories are likely to be involved, while the coleslaw will provide some 100-plus more, depending on the weight of mayonnaise or French dressing.

The baked beans provide plenty of protein, with a little more from the toast, but both also give a wealth of fibre;

something the hamburger has none of and the coleslaw only a little. The meal contains about 300 calories and also provides plenty of vitamins A and C.

2 *Two rounds of wholemeal sandwiches, filled with egg and salad, versus 8oz steak with mustard and radiccio (red lettuce).*

Both meals provide protein, but while the wholemeal version provides fibre from the bread too, lettuce isn't particularly fibrous. The sandwiches meal, provided you are mean with butter or margarine and don't add mayonnaise to the egg, contains about 460 calories, using 1 large egg. The steak, even if it's lean, contains about the same, but you may find it difficult to avoid adding chips! So the advantage of the sandwiches is fibre.

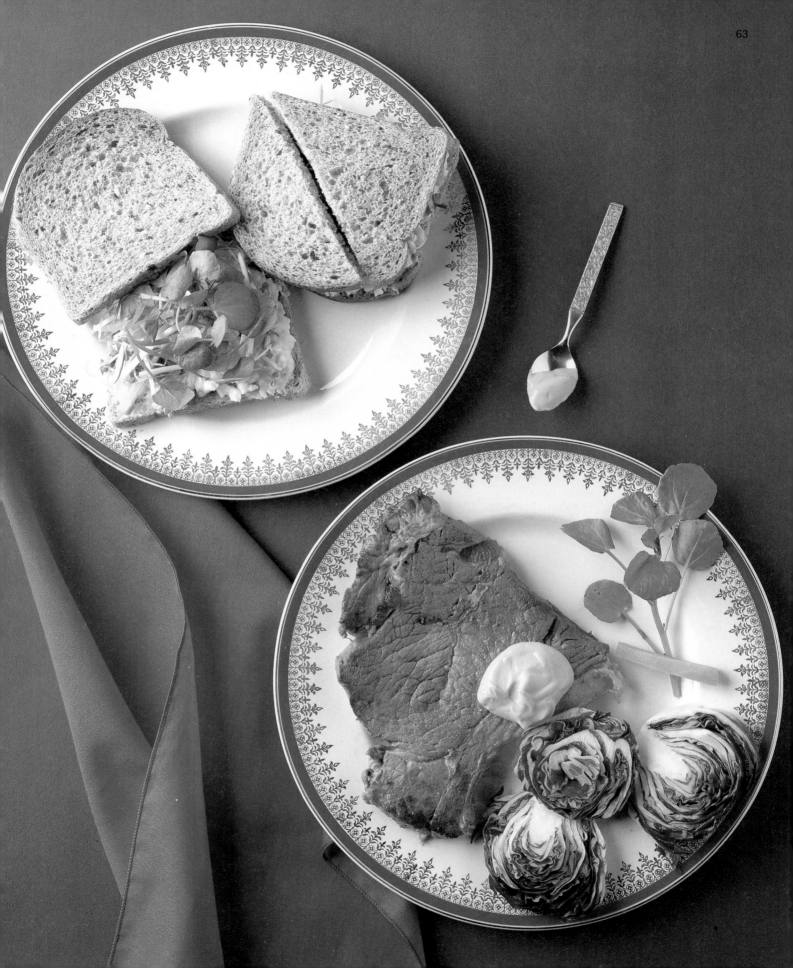

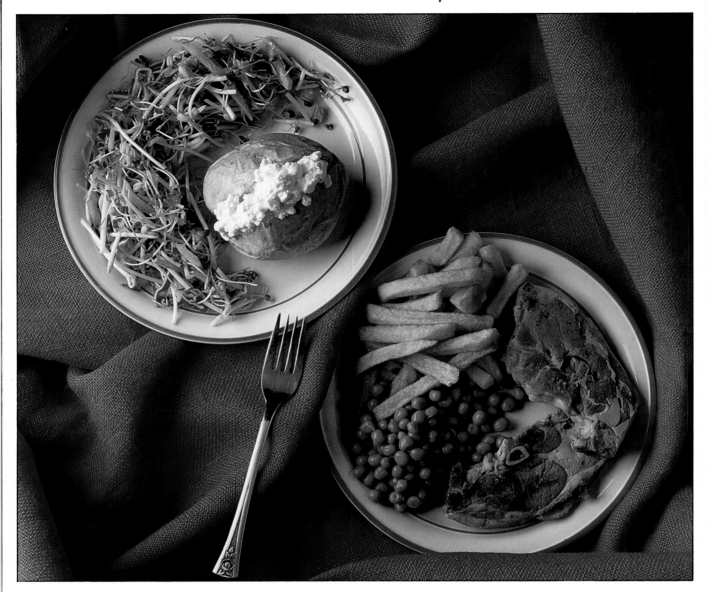

Above: potatoes aren't fattening – when compared to the meal with lamb chops; that plateful has less than half the calories.
Opposite: two pub lunches – and the shepherd's pie has less calories as well as less fat and more fibre, and more to eat.

3 *A large, 9oz baked potato filled with 2oz cottage cheese, and a generous plate of mixed salad, versus 7oz lamb chops with 4oz chips and 2oz peas.*

Because of the amount of fat on chops, this 'meat and two vegetables' meal carries around 500 calories for the meat, 30 for the peas and 280 for the chips! That makes about 810. The chips contain only a small amount of fibre, so the peas are the only good source. The potato – which many of us like to eat, but some imagine is too fattening – contains around 300 calories including cottage cheese and salad. It isn't as high in protein as lamb chops, but when you add in the cottage cheese and salad protein, you end up with a meal that provides about a quarter of an adult's total daily protein need, plus fibre from potato and salad. If you wanted extra protein, you

could add more cottage cheese for a 'lean' protein meal.

4 *A ploughman's lunch of 112g (4oz) Cheddar cheese, 40g (1½oz) French roll, 20g (¾oz) butter and 1 tbsp chutney, versus 200g (7oz) shepherd's pie with cauliflower, carrots and green beans.*

You may think of the first meal as 'light', but with this amount of cheese, you'll be getting about 2oz pure fat if you count the butter and, if the bread is white, virtually no fibre. The shepherd's pie meal has a potato topping, which is usually low fat and includes some fibre, plus all the fibre from the vegetables. It's considerably lower in calories, depending on vegetable portions and the proportion of fat in the meat; 400 calories versus about 640.

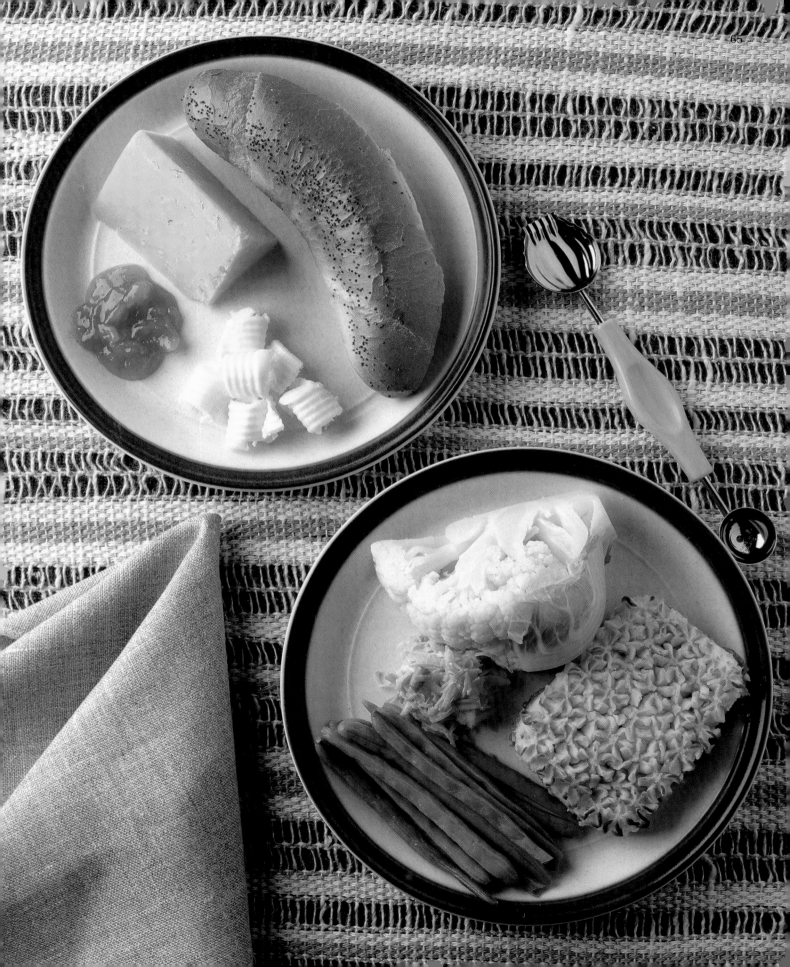

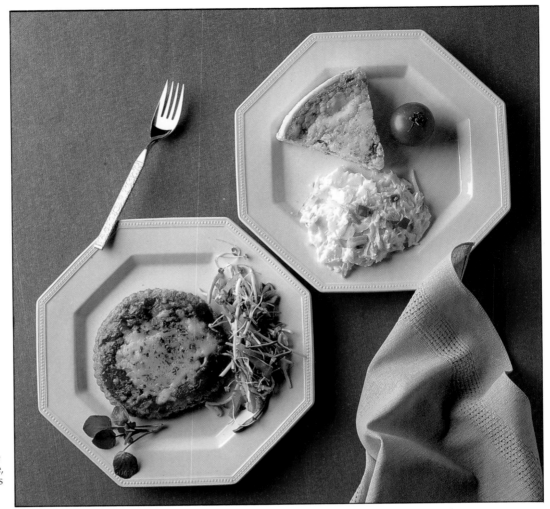

Right: quiche has a 'healthy' image, but is high in fat and calories. You're better off with the whole-meal pizza.
Opposite: "I just had a sandwich for lunch" can mean more calories, if you choose cheese (30% fat) on buttered bread, than a good plate of chicken, rice and vegetables. Brown rice, with its extra fibre, vitamins and minerals, scores over white bread, too.

5 *Two small rounds of toasted cheese sandwiches, with tomato and watercress, versus 4oz roast chicken with carrots, 3oz (cooked weight) brown rice and browned mushrooms.*

You might think the first meal is lighter, but because the bread is white, even the admirable tomato and watercress mean it's low fibre, with considerable fat from the cheese. The calorie count: about 500, allowing for 1½oz grated cheese and about ½oz butter. It's easy to spread butter liberally on hot toast and bought toasted sandwiches are often buttered on the outside, too.

The chicken meal has about 400 calories, allowing for 1 tsp oil to brown the mushrooms in – they contain so few calories, you can have as many as you want – and a generous helping of carrots. It will contain about 60 calories fewer if you don't eat the chicken skin, which carries most of the fat, which this meal has little of. The chicken meal provides two kinds of fibre, from the brown rice and the vegetables.

6 *Wholemeal pizza with mixed salad, versus quiche with tomato and mayonnaise coleslaw.*

The wholemeal pizza has more fibre than the quiche, because it's made with wholemeal flour, and it contains more vitamins and minerals, too. It also has less fat, because the bread dough used in pizza is low fat, while shortcrust pastry is about 30% fat. Quiche fillings are high in fat from milk, cheese, eggs and often bacon, too. The salad with the pizza isn't deluged in greasy mayonnaise (79% fat) like the coleslaw, and you actually eat more salad, so get more fibre from it. The pizza still provides enough protein, but mainly from the low fat wheat, plus cheese in topping. For the same calories as a 5oz piece of quiche (approximately 550 calories), you can eat an 8oz piece of pizza, or you could save some calories by eating the same amount. Every tablespoon of mayonnaise or a bought coleslaw adds about 100 calories, 80 of them from fat, to your meal.

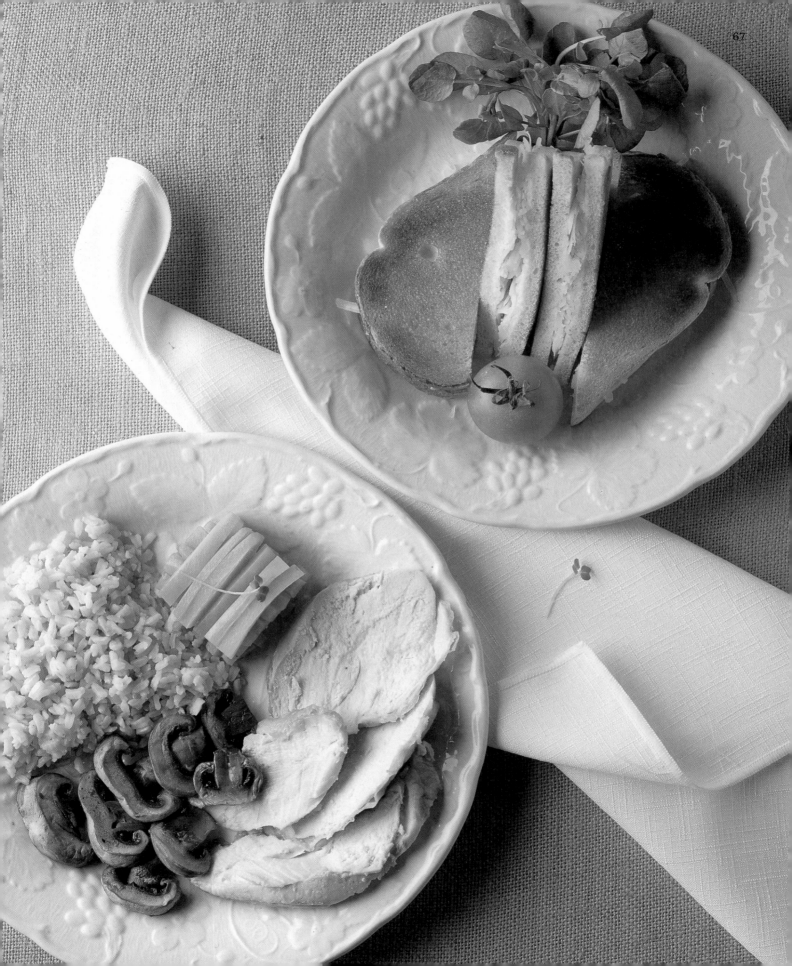

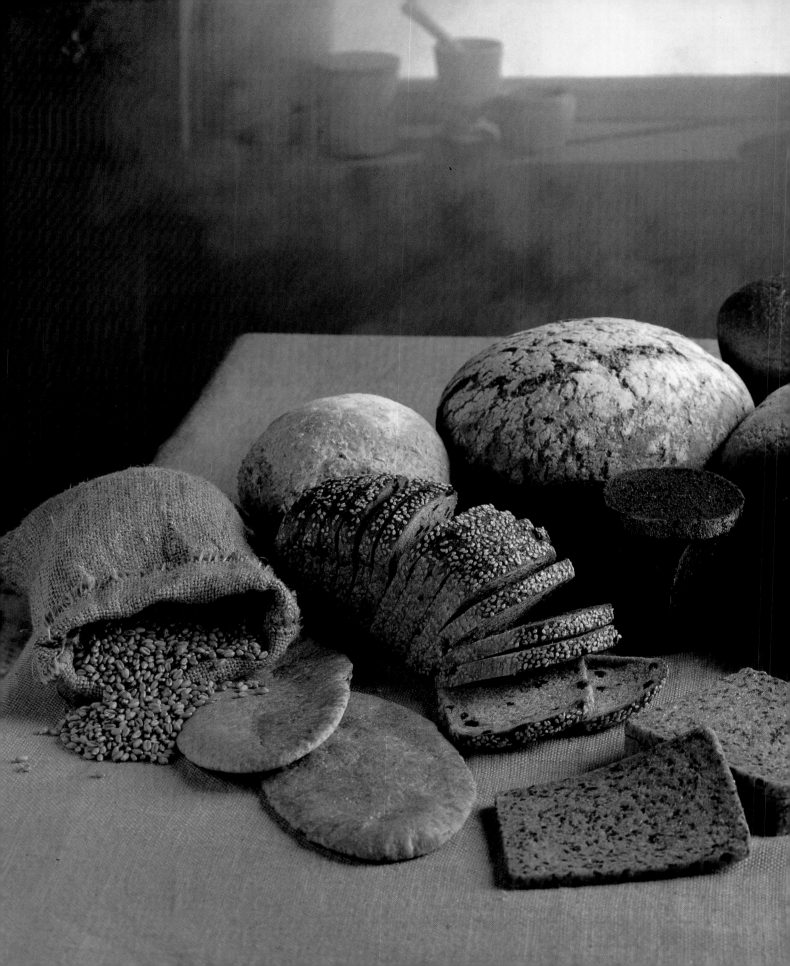

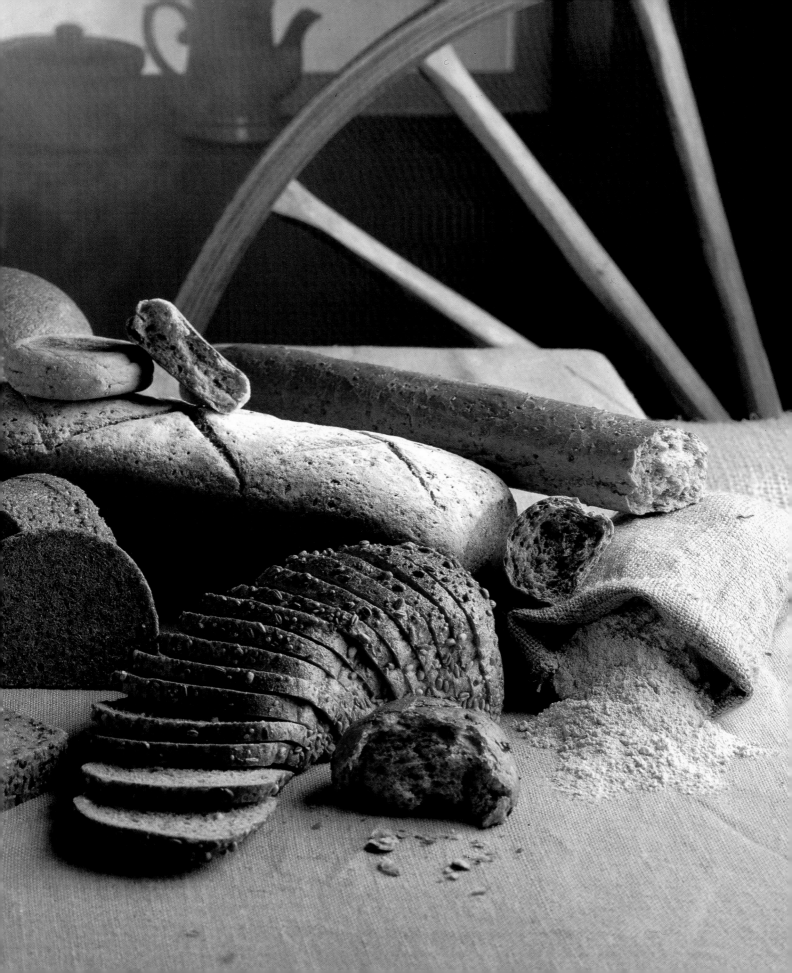

Bread – the Staff of Life

If you go into a supermarket or bakery, the choice of bread can be both delightful and confusing! Which is the healthiest?

All brown bread will contain more fibre than white, with Granary tm the next highest in fibre after wholewheat. All the same, brown bread may contain only about a third as much fibre as wholewheat, so the '100%' label indicating that the loaf is wholemeal or wholewheat is worth looking for. You're getting more B vitamins

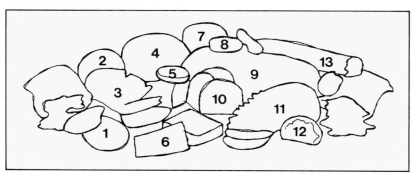

Key to bread photo, previous page: 1. wholemeal pitta bread; 2. brown soda bread; 3. wholemeal raisin-and-sesame cob; 4. round French country bread (made with little yeast and long rising time to give special tangy flavour); 5. black rye loaf; 6. pumpernickel slices with linseed; 7. Granary™ cob; 8. wheatmeal muffin; 9. long French brown bread; 10. rye and wheat pumpernickel; 11. Dr. Vogel mixed grain loaf; 12. Granary™ roll; 13. wholemeal French stick.

and more minerals too. Wholemeal bread also has slightly fewer calories, and if you are planning to increase your fibre intake by getting more of your protein from bread, this can add up to quite a substantial saving. If you usually eat 5 slices a day, changing to wholemeal will save about 30 calories, which over a year represents 3lb from your waistline. Even among wholemeal breads, you'll find a fascinating choice which is widening yearly: pumpernickel, sourdough and more.

Wheatmeal is another name used for brown but not wholemeal bread, and the term covers a wide range of breads which vary from almost white to almost wholemeal. Apart from the high fibre Granary loaf, you'll find mixed grain loaves, which may be as good as wholemeal in food value, but can't call themselves wholemeal because their ingredients include some not included in the legal definition of wholemeal, such as linseed or sunflower seed.

Wheat germ breads are made by adding back to white flour a larger amount of wheat germ than would naturally be there. This provides more B vitamins and vitamin E, some fibre – but less than Granary – and makes the bread slightly sweet. Wheatmeal 'soda' breads are raised with soda rather than yeast, from Irish traditions.

Pick the wholemeal loaf most often, but even the brown ones are better than white, and better than alternatives such as high fat quiches or pies.

What to Spread Bread may be low in fat, 'but what about the butter?', you may ask. It's certainly possible to unbalance your healthy bread by a high fat spread. Here's a choice of spreads to keep your bread healthy and unfattening:

Butter: you don't need to give it up, but use it sparingly, most easily done if you don't keep it too cold. Try keeping butter for the day in the week when you have most time to enjoy breakfast, but using other fats for other days and for cooking. It contains 205 calories per ounce. Unsalted or slightly salted types are preferable.

Soft margarine high in polyunsaturates: is the only margarine worth giving up butter for! It has the same 205 calories per ounce, but provides more of the fats the body really needs and has less tendency to raise the level of fat in the blood. However, you should still use this sparingly, choosing lower-fat spreads most of the time. You can bake well with this kind of margarine.

Low fat spreads: contain only half as much fat as either butter or margarine, approximately 105 calories per ounce. This makes them worth trying for taste; some contain more PUFAs than others but all are useful.

Sunshine spread: is a way of getting a more natural spread than margarine, which is always processed, and getting some taste of butter too! You just beat into some softened butter about half its weight of an oil very high in polyunsaturates, say sunflower or safflower. It will look odd at first, but when chilled again forms into an easy-to-spread consistency. You will probably need an electric beater to save on the hard work. It contains around 220 calories per ounce, so you don't save any calories but just produce a spread, mixing butter taste and PUFAs, without additives.

Smoothie: an unprocessed lower fat spread, made by mixing equal amounts of slightly softened butter or high PUFA margarine (no need to soften this), with low fat curd or cottage cheese (sieve the latter). It contains around 120 calories per ounce.

Curd and cottage cheese: both make good spreads for bread on their own, at around 36 or 30 calories per ounce respectively. In this case, make sure you get your polyunsaturates by using oils high in them for salads or cooking.

Other spreads: keep in mind that sandwiches don't have to have a spread before filling, providing the filling is moist.

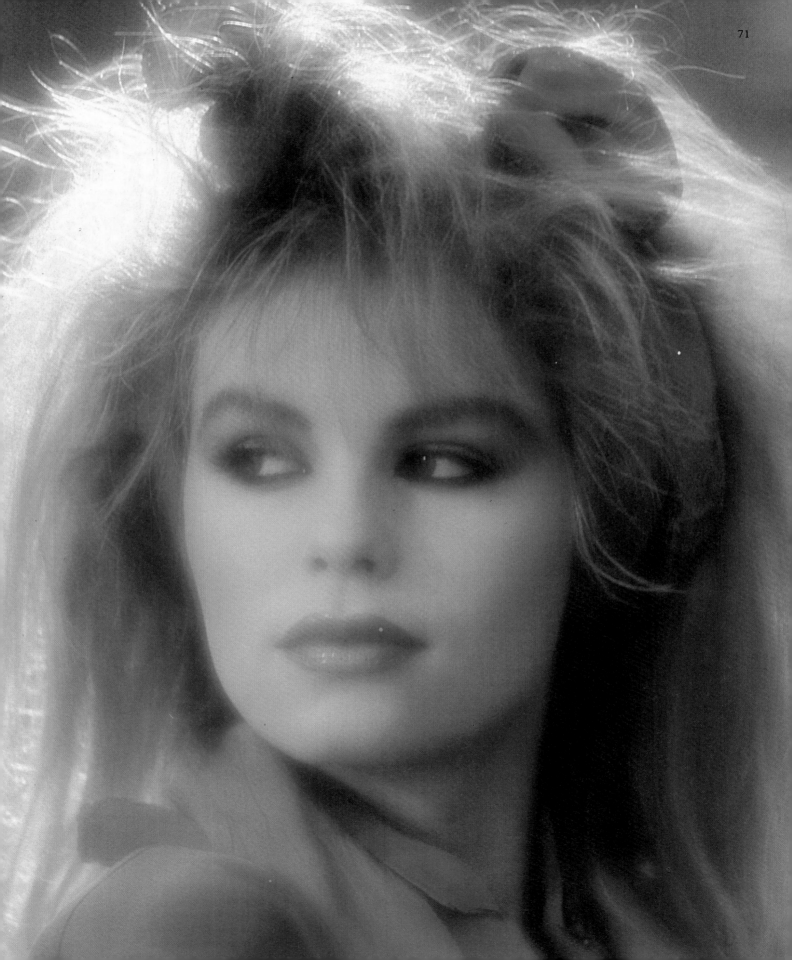

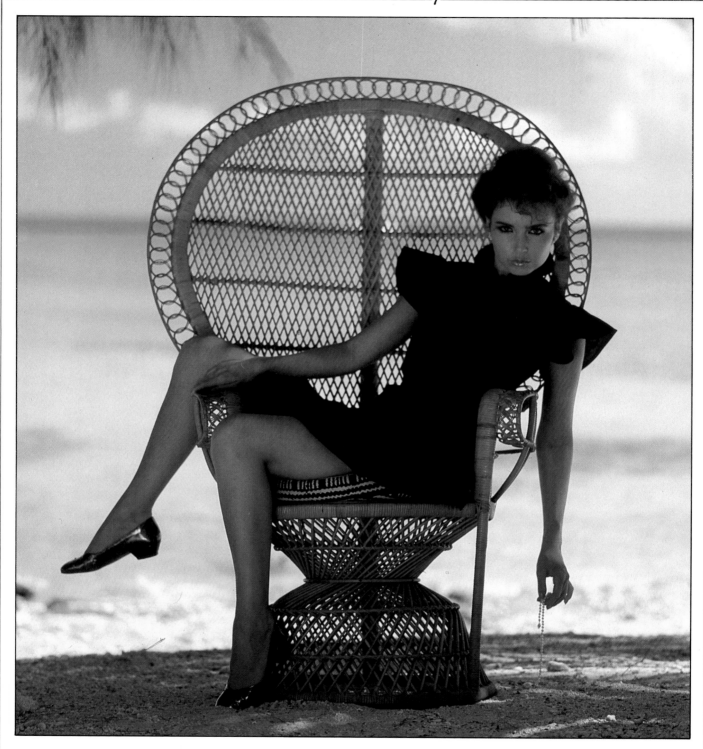

You are what you spread: see details on page 70. Clockwise from top: butter, soft margarine high in polyunsaturates, low-fat spreads sold in tubs, sunshine (butter-and-oil) spread, smoothie (butter-and-soft-cheese) spread, curd cheese and cottage cheese.

Try yeast extract, mashed bananas, mashed sardines and dried apricot purée, for instance, and skip the butter or margarine.

Other high fibre foods: as well as wholemeal bread include coconut, blackberry, sweetcorn, puffed wheat, prunes, dried apricots, blackcurrants, green beans, lentils, brown rice, beans, nuts, passion fruit,

and variations on the same foods i.e. unrefined cereals, dried fruit, berry fruit, dried beans and lentils, nuts.

How Much Fibre Do You Need? The ideal amount of fibre for good health is unknown, but for practical purposes, the target is at least 30 grams a day. This is about twice the fibre eaten in a typical Western

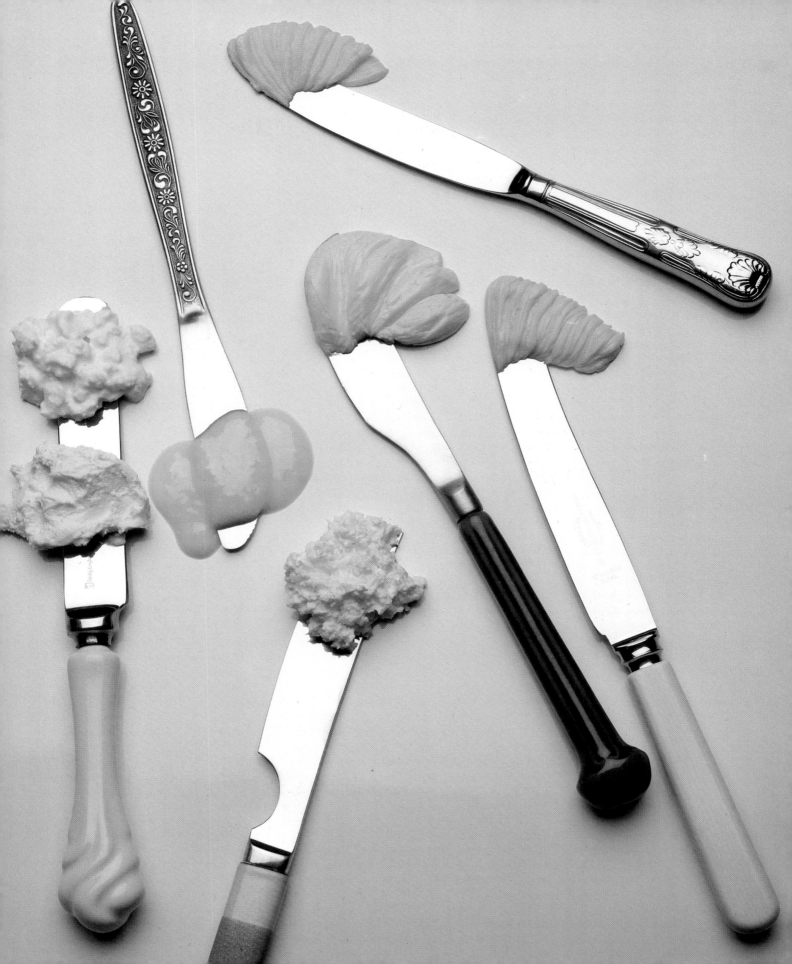

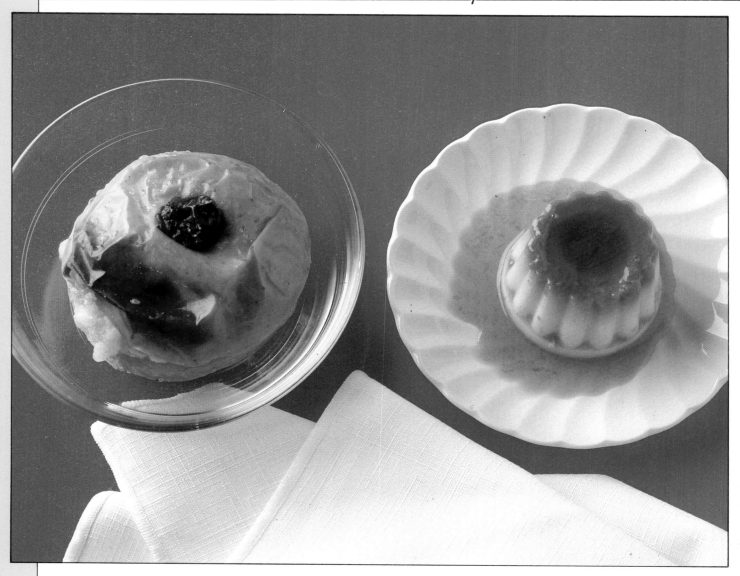

Fibre doesn't mean stringy! Above: high fibre baked apple versus no fibre caramel cream. Opposite: chili con carne (bean fibre) and high fibre peas and brown rice, versus low fibre white rice, no fibre chicken. Both delicious – so why not pick the fibre foods more often?

diet with white bread and little vegetables. However, it's not difficult to add fibre without adding bran from a packet.

Aim to have about 5 'fibre foods' a day at least, mixing the types. Here are some of the choices:

Wholemeal bread, fresh fruit,
bean salads, baked beans,
chilli con carne, unrefined breakfast
cereals,
porridge, crispbread,
brown rice, beansprouts,
banana, carrots,
humus, dhal (Indian spiced lentils),
dried fruit, vegetables, especially green
beans,
peas, sweet corn,
broad beans, nuts,
soft fruit, wholemeal pasta,
potato, large helping.

Here's an example of how keeping fibre in mind can produce a high fibre style of eating without you even noticing, compared to a low fibre meal.

High	Low
Chilli con carne	Chicken casserole
Brown rice	White rice
Celery	Cauliflower
Peas	

The low fibre menu contains virtually no fibre, except for the cauliflower. The high fibre menu includes all three types of fibre: from beans, in chilli, from brown rice and from vegetables, especially the peas. You certainly don't need to add bran to this style of eating.

Fibre in Pudding	*No Fibre*
Baked apple stuffed with minced dried fruit	Caramel dessert from shop

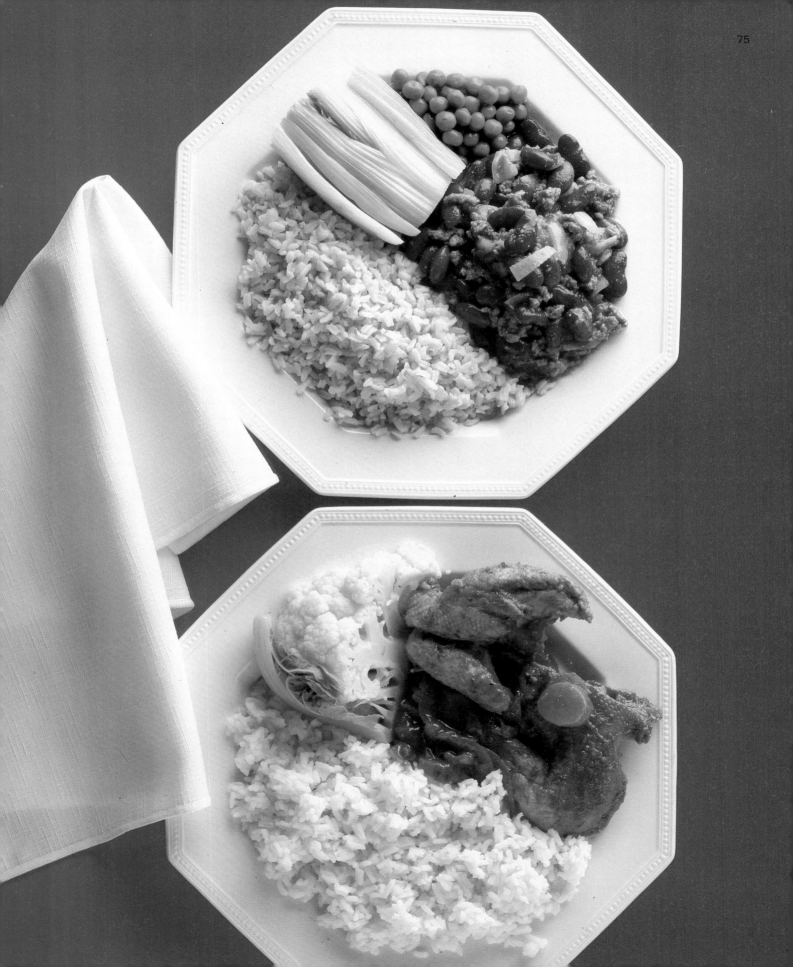

CHAPTER 6

Salt and a Healthy Diet

We all need some sodium, the main ingredient of table salt, but thanks to the amount added to foods in processing, and added by us in cooking or at table, the average person eats some 2 or 3 times as much as the level considered desirable. Excess salt can encourage high blood pressure in people who are vulnerable to this condition; which comes to some 1 in 4 or 5 of us at some time in our lives. High blood pressure isn't a disease in itself, but a warning signal that the heart is having to overwork and that we are more vulnerable to a heart attack, stroke or kidney illness. We are more likely to retain excess fluid, too.

Reducing salt can help bring blood pressure down, in a more natural way than taking drugs and without any side-effects. This is most easily done by reducing the number of processed foods that you use; if you read the ingredients labels of food packets, you'll find that almost all of them have added salt. Take-away foods also tend to be very salty.

Salt isn't the only influence on blood pressure; the amount of fibre, especially the kind of fibre in oats and beans, can have an effect, if you step it up. Eating less fat can also reduce blood pressure. Other factors: being too heavy encourages blood pressure to rise too high; smoking is linked with high blood pressure; lack of exercise is a bad influence and being under stress can push up blood pressure, at least temporarily.

If you say that it's easier to take drugs than to counter high blood pressure by natural means, remember that most people have to continue taking the drugs for the rest of their lives, and many experience unpleasant side-effects. It's healthier to get into the habit of eating less salt early in life; you won't miss the surplus provided you have some salt.

Eating Less Salt You can reduce the amount of salt you eat very quickly just by

Opposite: it's much easier to remove a little of the unnecessary heap of salt we eat than to face years of taking drugs to control the high blood pressure extra salt can encourage in many older people. Old age may seem a long way away, but the habit of taking too much salt can start trouble building up early. And it's a habit that most people can easily change, using only half as much.

using a salt pourer with a smaller hole, and not salting a plateful of food before you even taste it!

It's easy to dodge some of the most obvious salty foods, too: crisps, salted nuts, highly salted coated chicken or fish and other snack and take-away foods whose saltiness is outstanding.

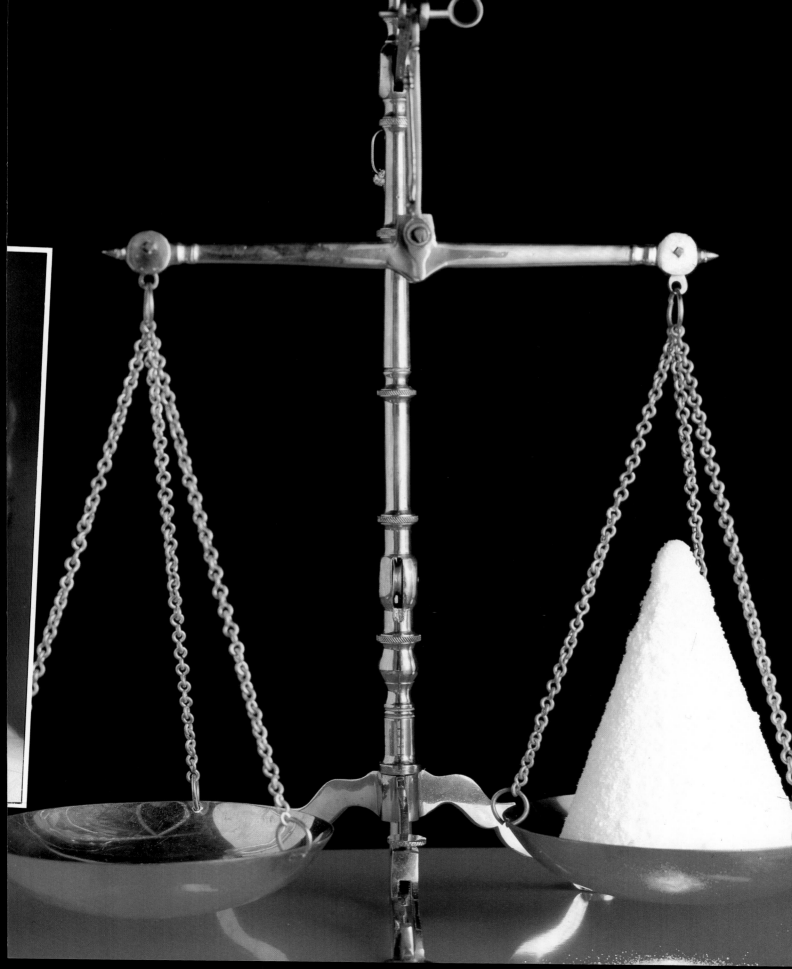

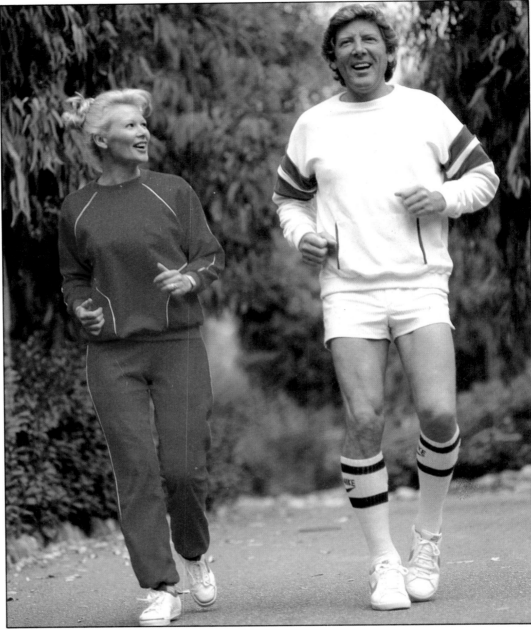

However much salt you may think you 'sweat off', you don't need as much as you eat. Clockwise from top right, opposite: yeast extract, Biosalt, mustard, salt substitutes, stock cubes, seaweed (sea vegetables), olives, Cheddar cheese, soya sauce, sesame salt, sea or rock salt crystals, herb salt, lemon juice.

Get out of the habit of automatically salting vegetables, rice or pasta cooking water; it's often unnecessary. If you cook vegetables only until they are just tender, not mushy, they'll have more of their own flavour and not need added salt. Let people add their own at table.

Choose unsalted or slightly salted butter instead of the saltiest, and flavour your cooking with other tastes instead of plain salt.

Here are some of the flavourings you can use to salt foods or give them flavour in other ways, so you don't need to use so much plain salt:

Yeast extract: is very salty, but it has a lot of other flavours too. So use it sparingly to flavour cooking or as a spread, and omit other salt from the recipe.

Biosalt: contains less sodium, because it is a mixture of minerals, all of which have some flavouring power. Still, use it sparingly.

Mustard: is a good salt substitute; if you make it up from powder it won't contain more than a trace of sodium. Made-up jars have added salt, but you can still end up with a lower-salt dish if you omit other salt from the recipe when using mustard.

Salt substitutes: contain other natural minerals, based on potassium, and virtually no sodium. They don't taste much like salt,

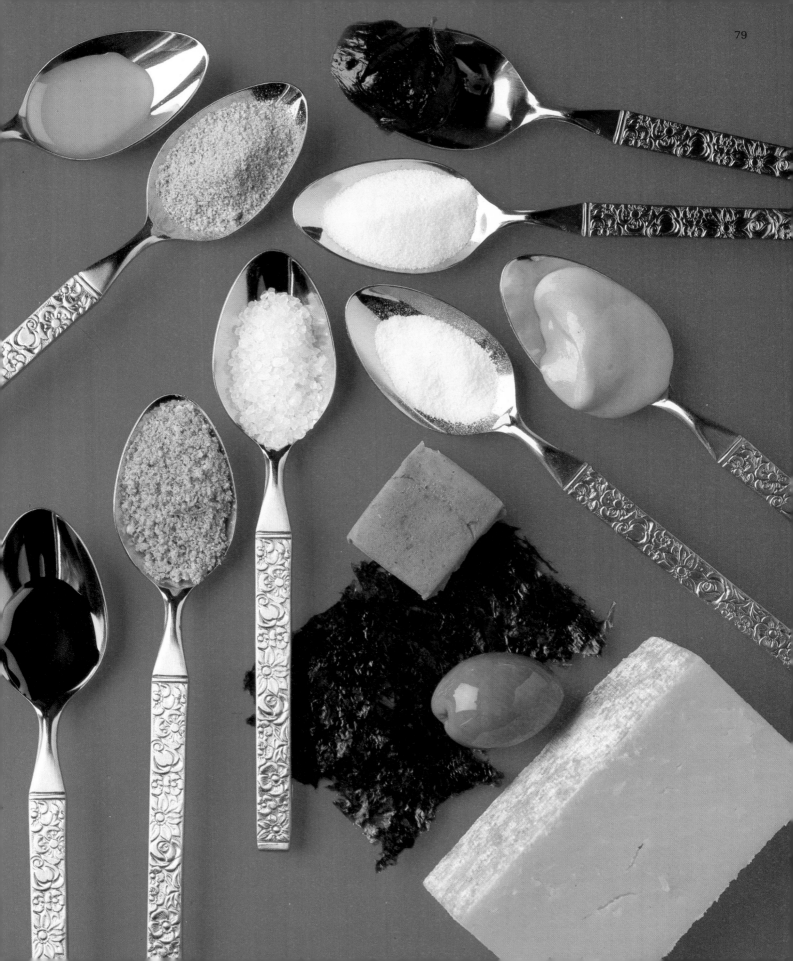

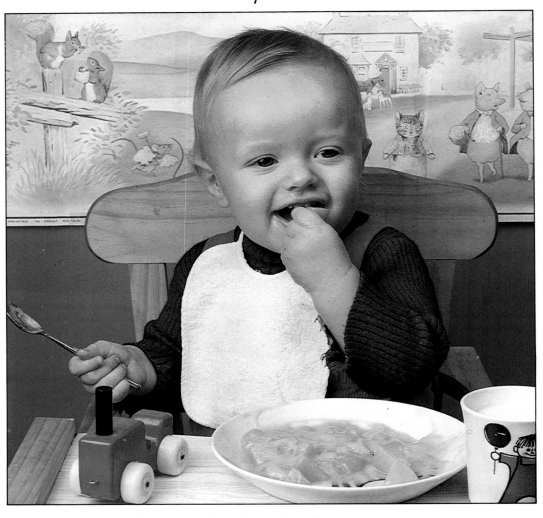

Right: added salt in food can be dangerous for babies, whose systems find it hard to cope with. To make baby food at home, remove child's portion from family meal before adding seasoning. But why add salt to the adults' food either? Apart from damage to health, excess salt can encourage fluid retention, blurring the clean lines of jaw and cheek with puffiness.

but try them to see whether you find they help you use less sodium. Anyone with a heart condition or on a low-potassium diet must check with their doctor before using these products.

Stock cubes: are usually very salty and are to be avoided, in favour of using your own cooking water from vegetables and meat as stock. You can buy low-salt stock cubes from health food stores. If you use stock cubes, omit other salt from recipe.

Nori: sheets of crisp, paper-thin seaweed from Japan with a naturally high salt content give flavour from other minerals. Use chopped nori or other cooked seaweed instead of salt to flavour meals.

Olives: are preserved in salty brine. So if you use them in pizza or other dishes, leave out any other salt.

Cheddar cheese: like almost all cheese, has a lot of salt added when it's made, as well as some natural sodium in milk. As it's high in fat too, use sparingly to replace salt in savouries, choosing the strongest-flavour type so you get more flavour with less cheese.

Soya sauce: is a salty Chinese and Japanese flavouring. Use sparingly; it will give you more taste than salt alone, so you need not use much.

Sesame salt: has only about half the sodium of ordinary salt, because it's mixed with toasted, crushed sesame seeds which contribute their own special flavour.

Sea salt: contains other useful minerals, especially iodine, which table salt doesn't have unless it's labelled 'iodized'. But it's still mainly sodium, so use as reluctantly as ordinary salt. You may find it easier to use less if you grind it each time in a salt mill.

Herb salt: has less sodium because it's mixed with powdered, dried herbs and vegetables. So if you use it like salt, you'll be getting extra flavour with less sodium. Use sparingly, unless you pick the type with no salt, only the vegetables.

Lemon juice: is the ideal salt substitute: it adds flavour, vitamin C and almost no sodium to food. Use freely, especially from fresh lemons.

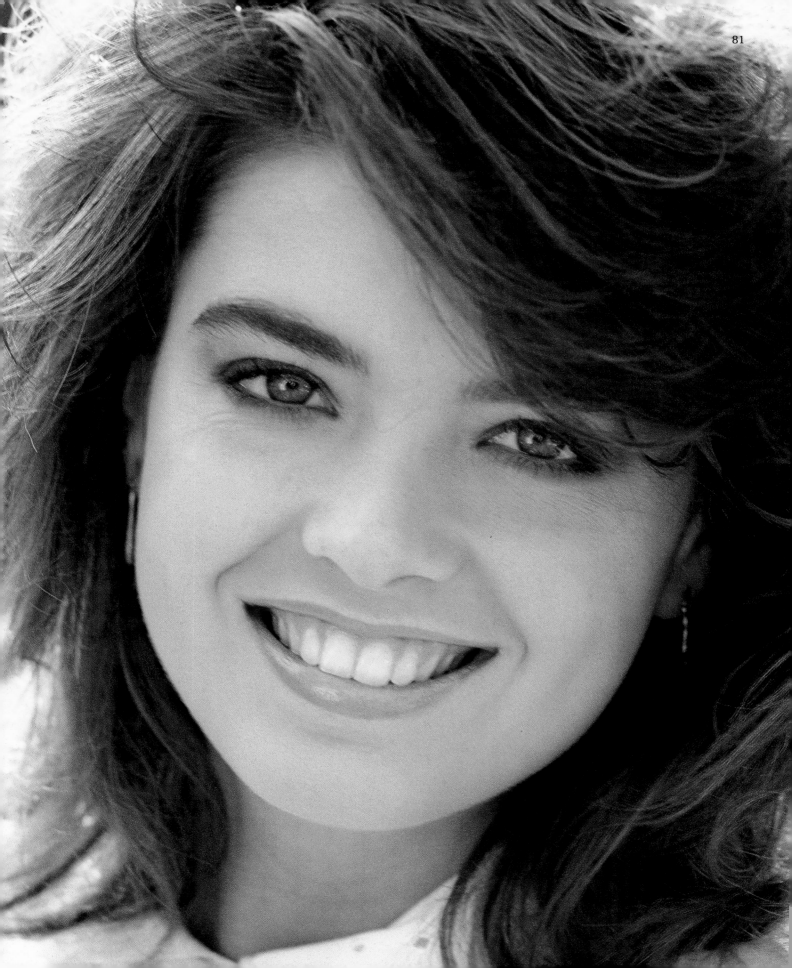

CHAPTER 7

Fresh Food and a Healthy Diet

Fruit and vegetables are our sole source, apart from milk and liver, of vitamin C (ascorbic acid). It's essential for many reasons, which can be summed up as protecting the body from vulnerability to infection and helping it recover if it does succumb.

Vitamin C is barely stored by the body, so it's important to eat some virtually every day. Vegetables are just as good sources as fruit, provided you pick at least some of them as leafy greens and eat a good proportion in salads, as even careful cooking causes some vitamin C loss.

When cooking either fruit or vegetables, the rules for keeping the best flavour *and* vitamin and mineral value are:

1 Only expose the cut or peeled surfaces to air for as short a time as possible. So don't cut or shred produce hours before it's going to be cooked or eaten.

2 Don't soak prepared produce, as vitamins and minerals will dissolve into the liquid. For the same reason, prefer methods

Eating plenty of fruit and vegetables – at least 2 or 3 helpings every day – gives the body plenty of the materials it needs to keep skin, hair, eyes and nails in good condition. And you can eat plenty of it while staying slim. But careless cooking can remove many of the vitamins and minerals from the food – so make the small effort to keep the goodness in.

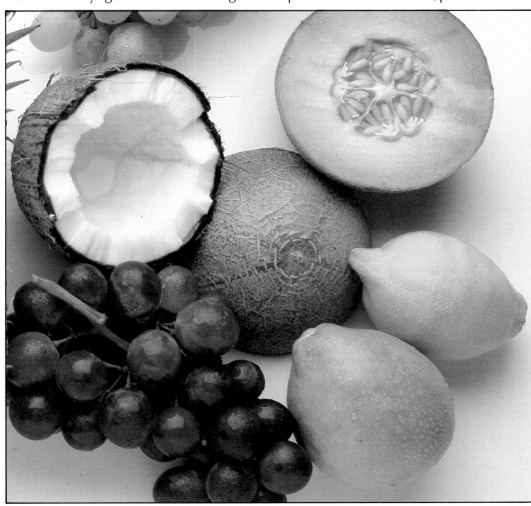

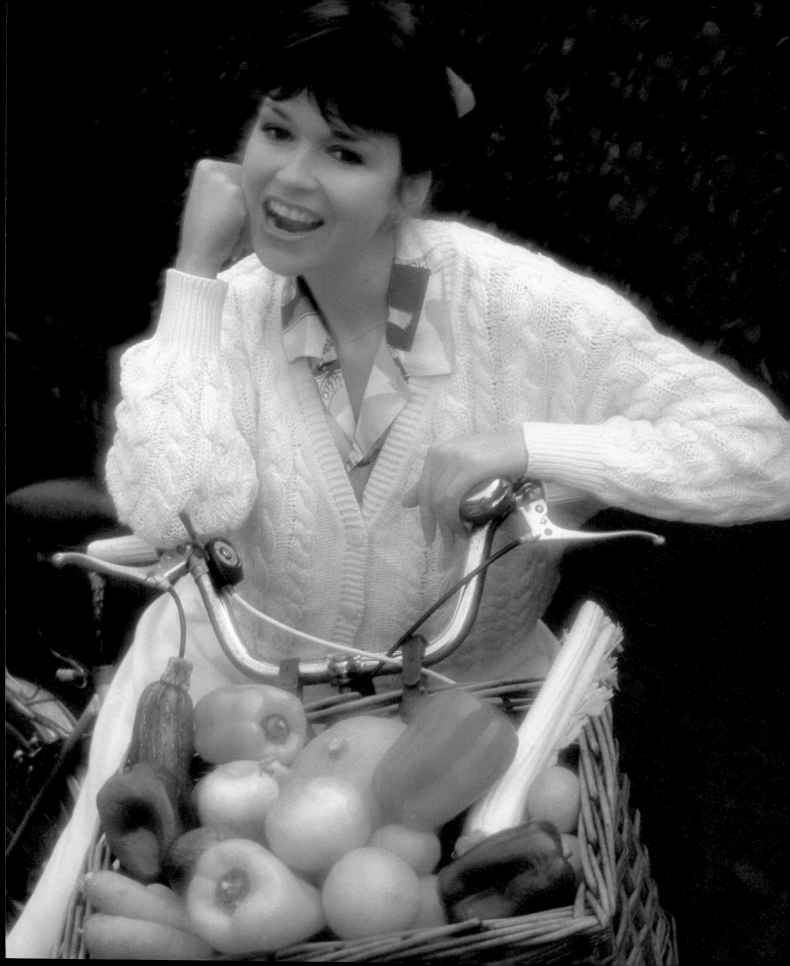

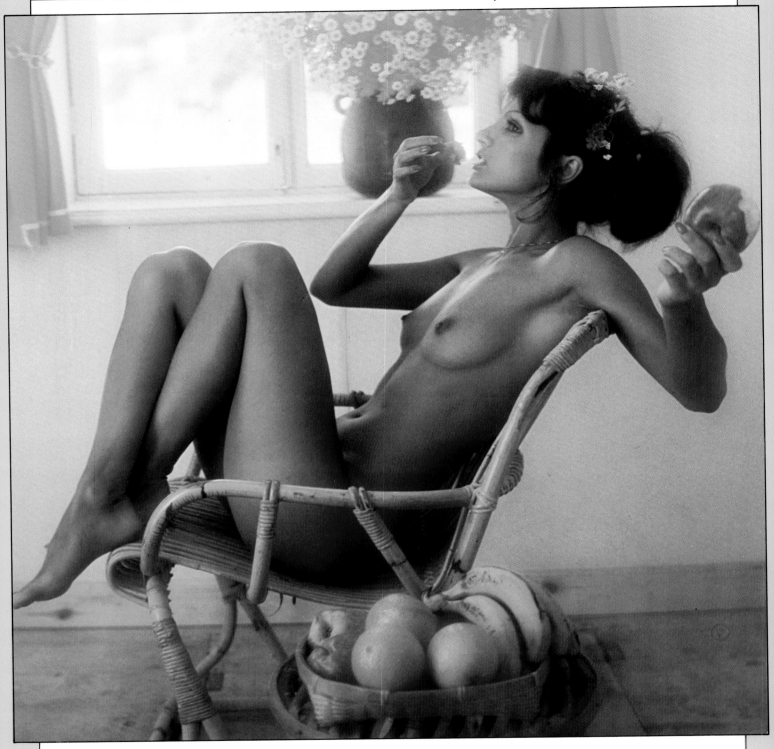

of cooking using no water, or the minimum: steaming, pressure cooking (a version of steaming), microwave cooking, or 'conservative' cooking, where you put only half a cup of water in a pan, boil it, add the vegetables, cover tightly and cook over a low-to-medium heat for several minutes. This is a 'half-steaming' method, where most of the vegetable barely touches water and little liquid is left at the end.

Any liquid left after cooking vegetables is worth keeping for the stock jug. It not only adds flavour to soups, casseroles or sauces, but also means you 'regain' some minerals and vitamins which may have dissolved in it.

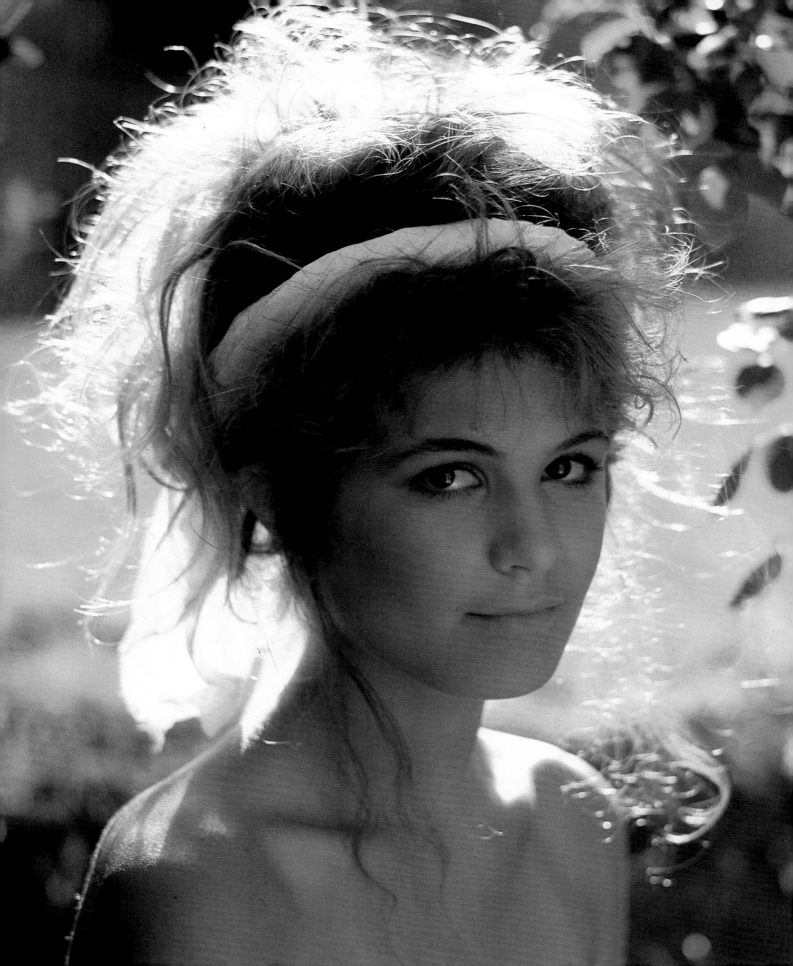

Below: vegetables are even more valuable than fruit, but use both. Yellow, red and orange types like carrot and pepper tend to be richest in vitamin A; leafy greens and citrus fruit, peppers and strawberries are top for vitamin C, but they are all good – and so delicious to eat, too.

3 Cook produce for the minimum of time. This reduces vitamin loss and keeps texture and flavour good, minimising the need for added butter or salt to make the produce enjoyable.

4 Avoid keeping vegetables hot, which causes substantial vitamin loss. Only start cooking them when everyone's at table.

5 If you want to use ready-prepared vegetables or fruit, frozen produce has a higher food value than tinned. If using tinned, use the liquid in cooking to regain minerals dissolved in it.

Aim to have fresh food with every meal, from fruit at breakfast time, to a salad as a daily habit, to snacks of raw carrots or bananas. Fruit and vegetables can be good 'convenience foods', because salads are easy to make and fruit can be eaten wherever you are.

Apart from their vitamin C, fresh produce is a major source of vitamin A in carotene form. This is richest in yellow and orange vegetables and fruit, together with leafy green vegetables. Leafy green vegetables also provide the best sources of folic acid (a

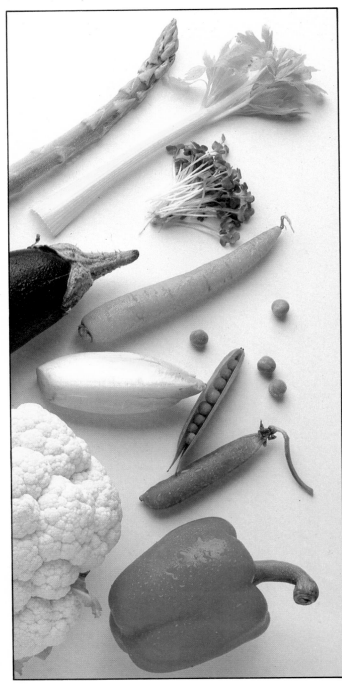

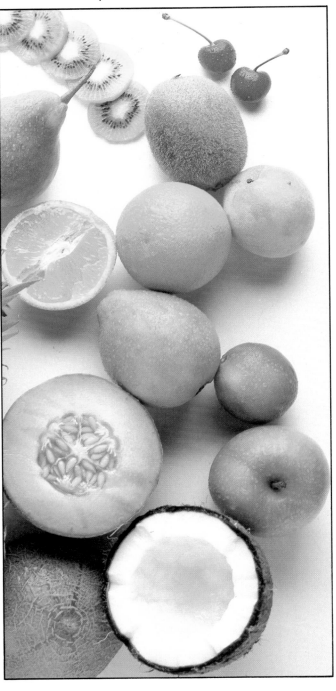

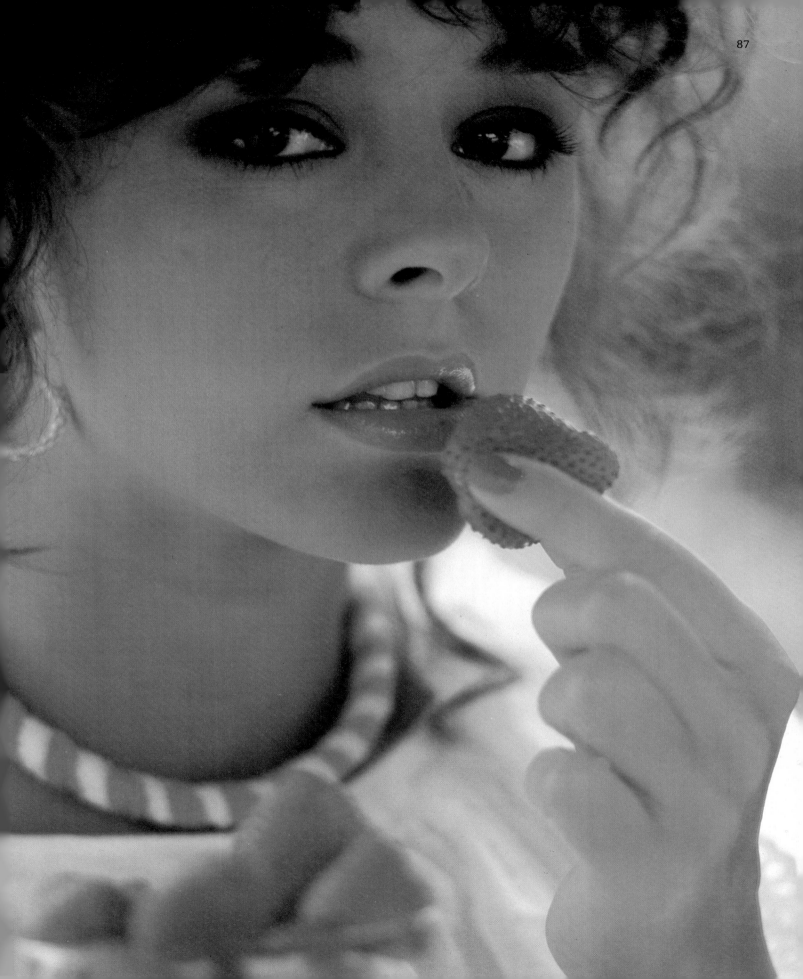

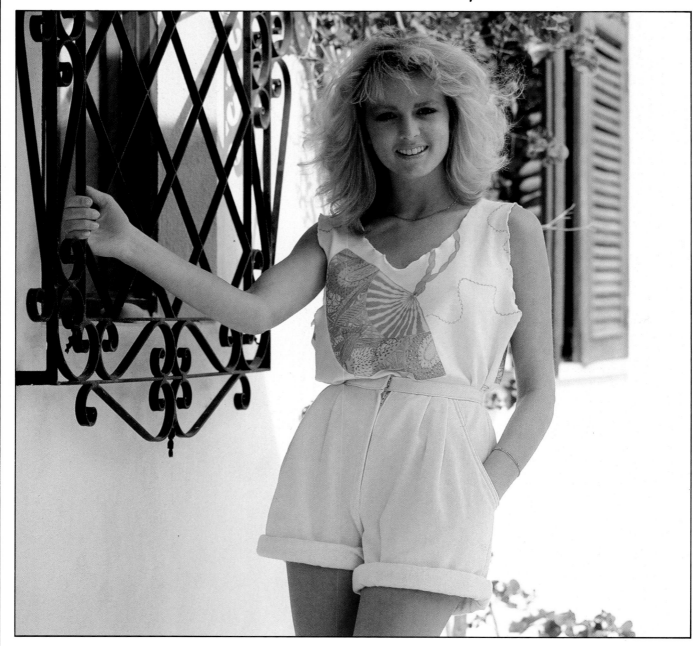

Think of yourself as someone special, worth feeding with the fresh and natural foods that will nourish you best. Don't see food as unimportant fuel, and eat the first food that comes to hand. You'll enjoy food – and life – more if you like yourself too much to fill up on 'junk'.

constituent of the vitamin B complex), vitamin E, vitamin K and a variety of minerals, including iron and calcium. This makes them particularly important, more so than fruit, and most useful of all if you don't want to eat much meat or milk products, which are the alternative and richest sources of iron and calcium respectively.

Leafy greens that are eaten raw, such as mustard and cress, celery leaves, shredded green cabbage (white is not so nutritious), watercress or alfalfa sprouts, are especially valuable because no food value is lost in cooking. Aim to eat leafy greenstuff at least once daily.

On top of all this, fruit and vegetables supply fibre, giving a satisfying bulk to meals without too many calories. Their rich variety of colours and flavours is vital to good cooking and means that you don't have to rely on high-fat butter, cream or oil to make food look and taste good. Make them a major part of your shopping list and keep them for as short a time as possible. Store vegetables in the refrigerator for crisp freshness: heat, light and exposure to air on cut surfaces are the major enemies of their freshness and food value.

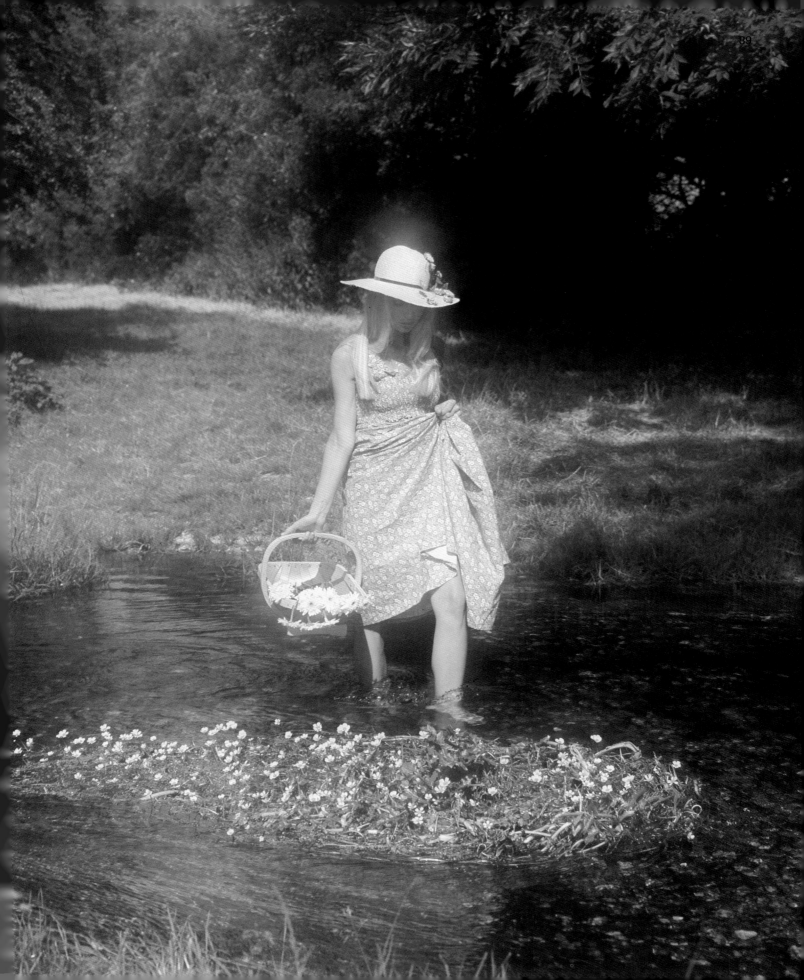

CHAPTER 8

The Healthy way to Lose Weight

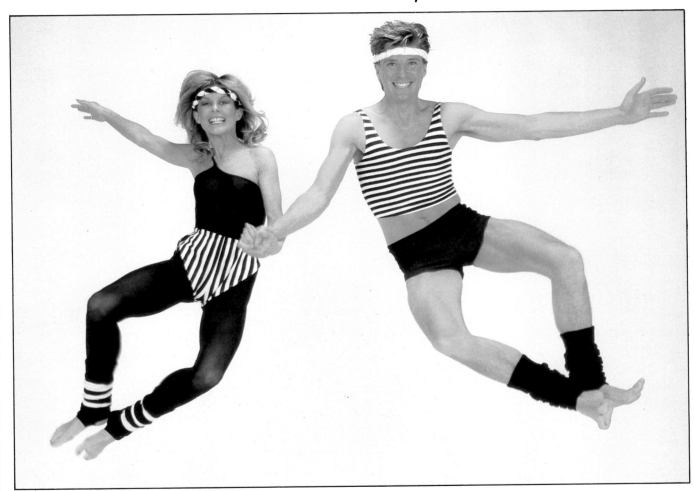

Why carry suitcases around with you – in the shape of excess poundage? It's nice to travel light, without wanting to be skinny. Keeping active while you lose weight makes the job much easier.

Follow this four-week eating plan for a sleeker, livelier you.
Being skinny isn't fashionable any more. Now the aim is to be in good shape; firm rather than frail. Beauty is the gleam of hair, skin and smile that comes from health. Give yourself the glossy good looks that come from the inside. The diet provides around 1,400 calories a day; more than the typical weight loss diet, less than the average woman's daily intake. If you know you find it hard to maintain a neat shape, trim the diet as suggested later.

Team the meal plan with 30 minutes of exercise each day. It'll not only firm up your shape, but also act as a mood-booster. If you feel lethargic, exercise can improve your energy level, which is another essential for good looks and success. If you feel tense or restless, exercise can help you relax. It can also help you stick to your eating plan. How? When you become more aware of your body, through sport or movement, you'll find you're keener to keep it in peak form by eating well. Also, when you keep active, you have less time

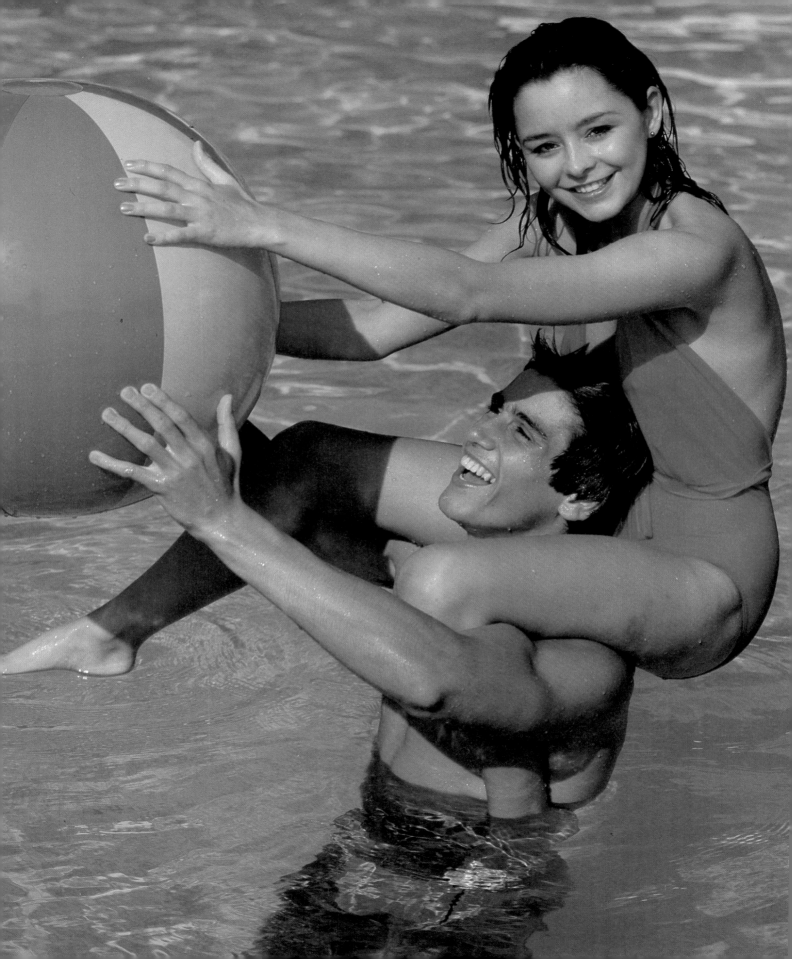

to be tempted towards the wrong foods.

This eating plan is different from other diets because its first aim is vitality; foods that give you best value-for-calorie are packed into it. Feeling good stops you eating for comfort when depressed, too. The foods that don't earn their keep with the meal plan through not having the right food to hand. To protect vitamins, keep all your vegetables cool and dark in the 'fridge'. Invest in the vitality foods; you'll save overall because you won't be spending money on soft drinks, sweets or take-away snacks.

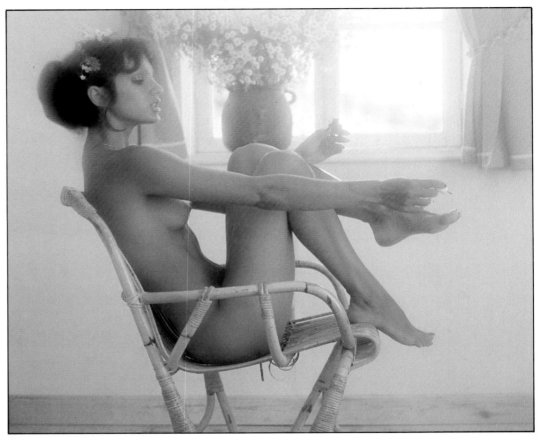

Beautiful bodies, above and opposite, should inspire you, and not make you give up because yours is so much fatter! We're all individuals, and there are many different body shapes which are beautiful, as great painters have proved. Find a model you are content with that's close to your figure type – then work gradually towards your target. It's better to change slowly and keep the weight off than to crash diet, then crash gain!

food value are booted out. If you find you've eaten the wrong thing one meal, don't worry, or give up. Just go back to the plan and notice how well you feel when you stick to it. You don't need to check this diet with your doctor unless you are under treatment for an illness.

Choose one breakfast, one light meal and one main meal every day. You don't have to try all the meals, but don't eat the same thing every day. Variety improves your chances of getting every vitamin or mineral you need.

If you don't usually eat breakfast, a style of eating like this may make you feel hungrier in the morning. If you don't eat breakfast, keep fruit and a made-up tub of one of the cereal or stewed fruit breakfasts handy for mid-morning, when you may otherwise be drawn to chocolate or bun!

Shop in advance, so that you don't give up

Measure out your daily allowance of spread and milk, so you know how much you are eating. It's useful to weigh out portions of other foods until you can judge by looking how large a 4oz potato is, for instance.

Your 28-Day Plan
Repeat the cycle 4 times.

Daily allowances
✱ 15g (½oz) butter, margarine high in polyunsaturates or other spread (105 calories). You can also use low fat spread, saving half these calories, but choose a type with a reasonable level of vegetable oils for PUFAs, e.g. mix soft margarine high in PUFA half and half with cottage cheese.
✱ 285ml (½ pint) skim milk (about 110 calories)
✱ Vegetables from 'free' list
✱ Drinks from 'free' list

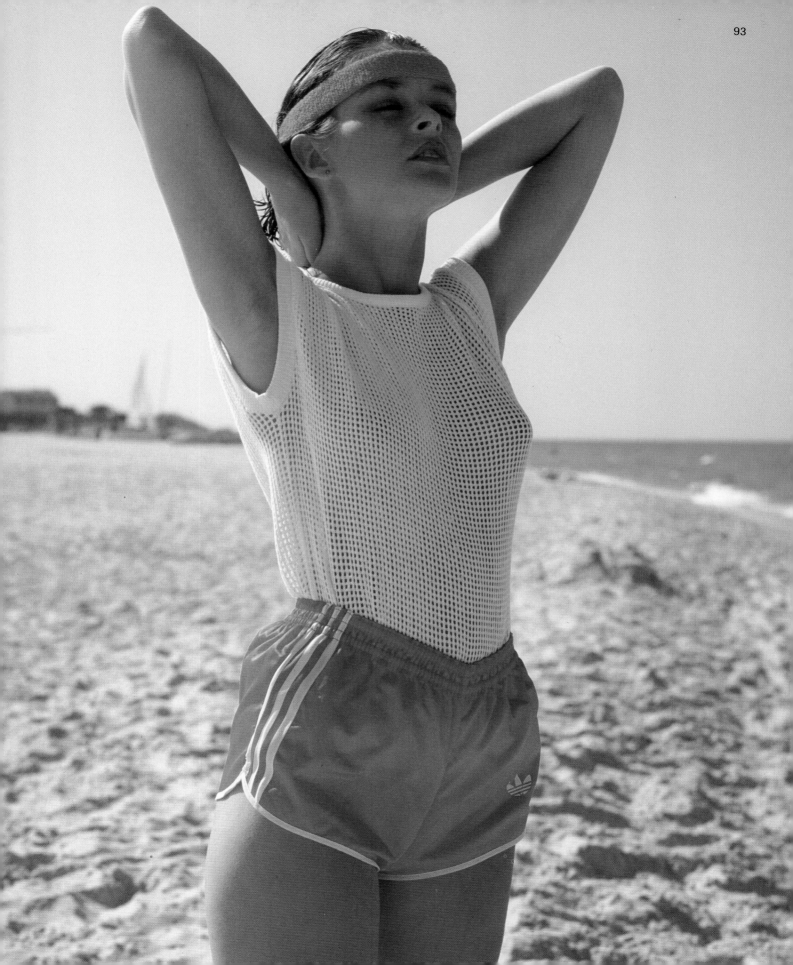

Breakfast Choices

1 *Total Calories 288*	*Approx. Cals.*	*Main food value*
1oz breakfast cereal, wholegrain such as muesli, unsugared brand	105	protein, fibre, B vitamins, E, minerals
1 apple (4oz approximately)	50	fibre, minerals
¼ pint unsweetened fruit juice or extra skim milk (not allowance)	50	vitamin C, minerals especially potassium or protein, B vitamins, calcium
2 tsp wheat germ (½oz)	40	protein, vitamins B and E, minerals, high-PUFA oil
1 tsp chopped nuts (¼oz)	43	high-PUFA oil, protein, B vitamins, minerals
drink from allowance, e.g. coffee	–	

N.B. Soak muesli in liquid overnight. In the morning, grate in apple and nuts, stir in wheat germ.

Below: breakfast 1: plenty to eat, thanks to soaking muesli overnight. Decaffeinated coffee.

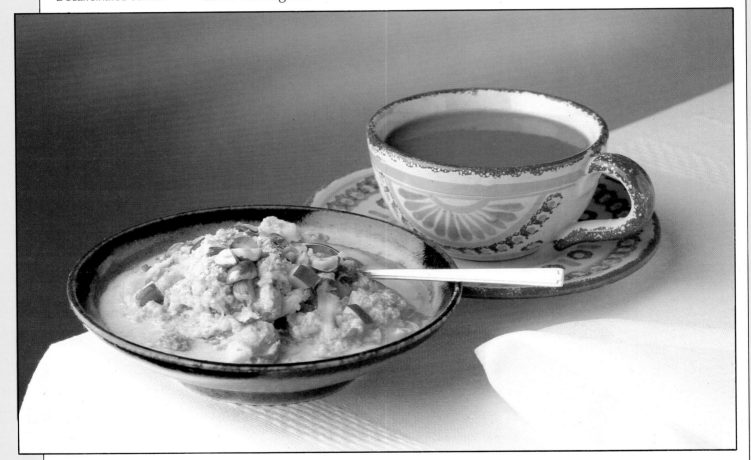

Right: breakfast 2: beautiful food is more satisfying, and no one can complain that this breakfast takes too long to make. Peppermint tea – or try limeflower for a morning boost.

2 *Total Calories 225*	*Approx. Cals.*	*Main food value*
10oz any fruit but banana	120	vitamins, minerals, fibre
5oz unsweetened low fat yogurt	75	protein, calcium, B vitamins
1 tsp clear honey	30	trace minerals
drink from allowance, e.g. peppermint tea	–	

N.B. Chop fruit or slice. Mix yogurt with honey.

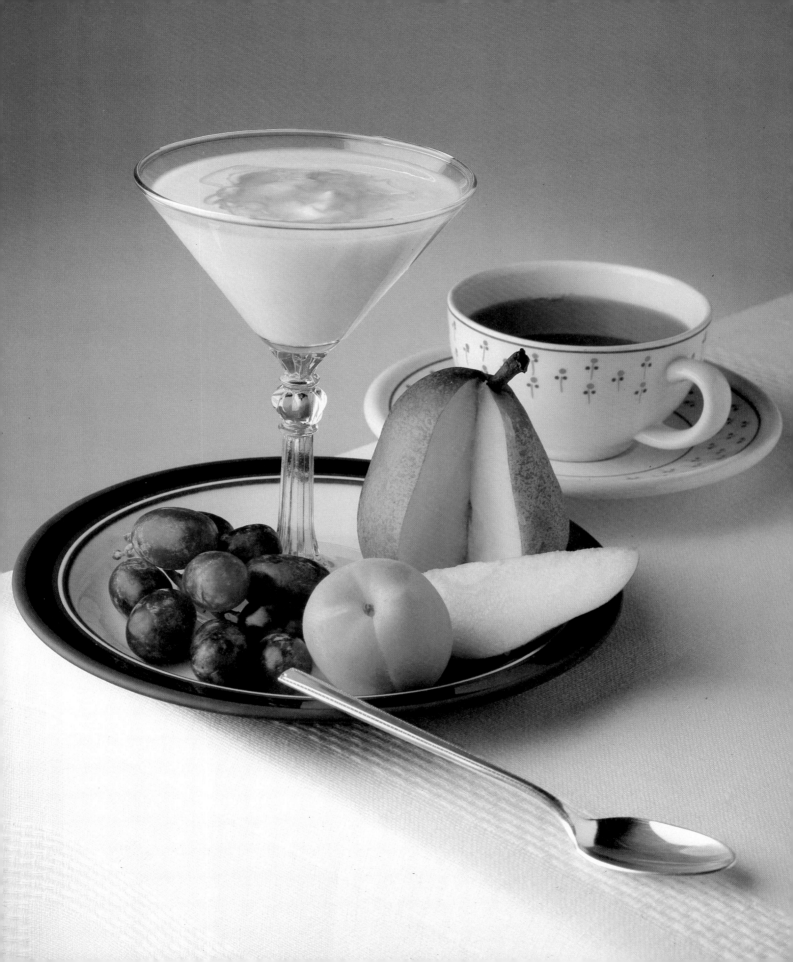

3 Total Calories 262	Approx. Cals.	Main food value
1 large boiled egg	90	protein, vitamins, iron, 13% fat
2 slices wholemeal 'soldiers'	122	protein, fibre, vitamins, minerals
spread from allowance	–	
1 piece of fruit (e.g. 4 oz apple)	50	fibre, minerals
drink from allowance, e.g. weak China tea	–	

N.B. Use as little salt as possible on egg.

Below: breakfast 3. Choose 'real' 100% wholemeal bread, not halfway-house 'brown' or 'wheatmeal', for the full benefit of fibre, vitamins and minerals. China tea.

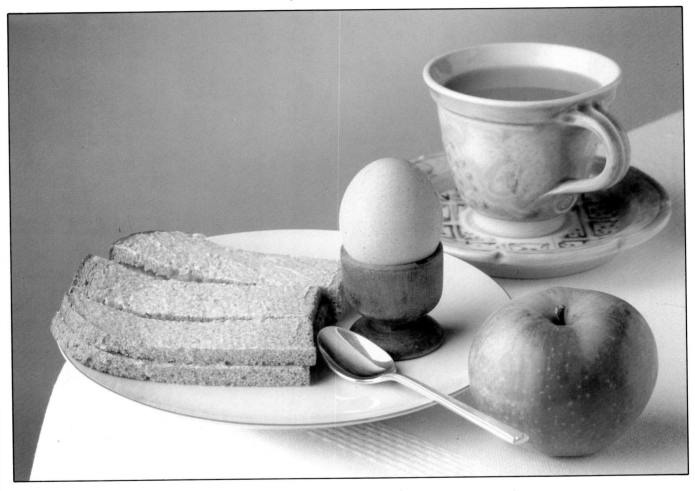

4 Total Calories 287	Approx. Cals.	Main food value
Fresh and dried fruit salad: 2oz stewed dried fruit, mixed	106	fibre, iron, other minerals
8oz fresh fruit, chopped	96	vitamins, especially C, and minerals, fibre
juice from stewing fruit	–	
2 tsp coarse bran	neg.	fibre
2 tsp wheat germ	40	protein, B and E vitamins, minerals, high-PUFA oil
3 tbsp (3oz) low fat yogurt	45	protein, B vitamins, calcium
drink from allowance, e.g. lemon barley water	–	

Opposite: breakfast 4 – a perfect starter to a summer's day. Vary the fruit as much as you like to suit what's in season and good value. Home-made lemon barley water is a wonderfully refreshing drink. (Boil 1oz barley and rind of 1 lemon, simmer for a few minutes, pour into jug, cool. Add juice of lemon and honey to taste. Strain and chill.)

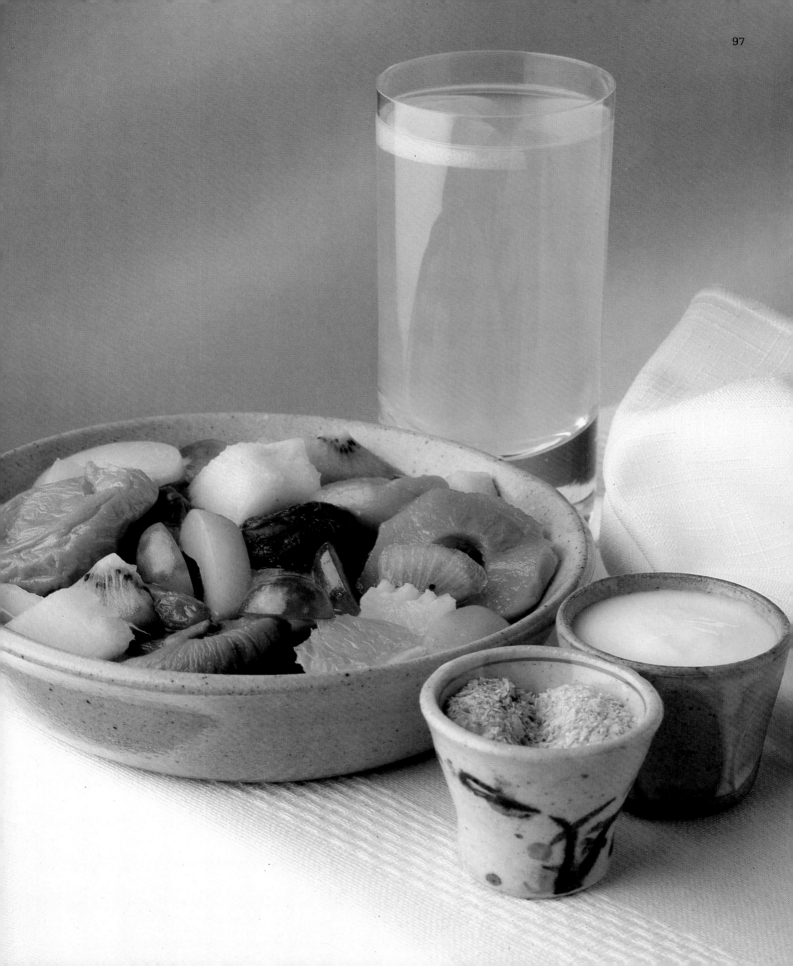

Below: breakfast 5. For a change, use grilled mushrooms instead of tomatoes, and other kinds of fresh fruit. You can add tea – herb or regular – without sweetening, if you like.

5 Total Calories 207	Approx. Cals.	Main food value
4 halves grilled tomato	20	vitamins A and C, fibre, minerals
spread from allowance	–	
1 slice wholemeal toast (1¼oz)	77	protein, fibre, B and E vitamins, minerals
5oz pear	60	fibre, minerals
5oz glass buttermilk	50	protein, calcium, B vitamins

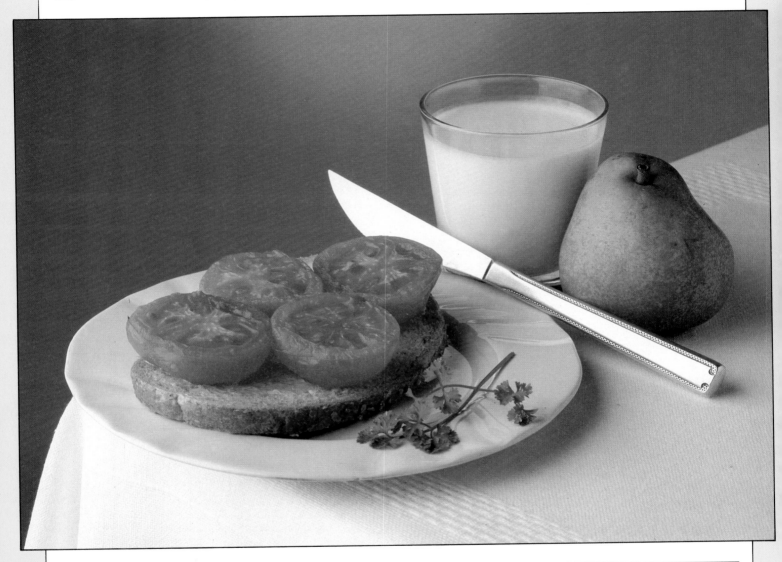

Opposite: breakfast 6. Ideal for a frosty morning, porridge really warms you up, with a hot glass of tea. The dried fruit can be mashed into the porridge to give extra sweetness.

6 Total Calories 365	Approx. Cals.	Main food value
Porridge using 1½oz oats	165	protein, fibre, B vitamins, minerals
¼ pint extra skim milk	50	protein, calcium, B vitamins
2oz dry weight prunes and apricots, stewed	100	fibre, minerals
1 piece fresh fruit, not banana	50	vitamin C (not particularly high in apples), minerals, fibre
drink from allowance, e.g. rosehip tea	–	

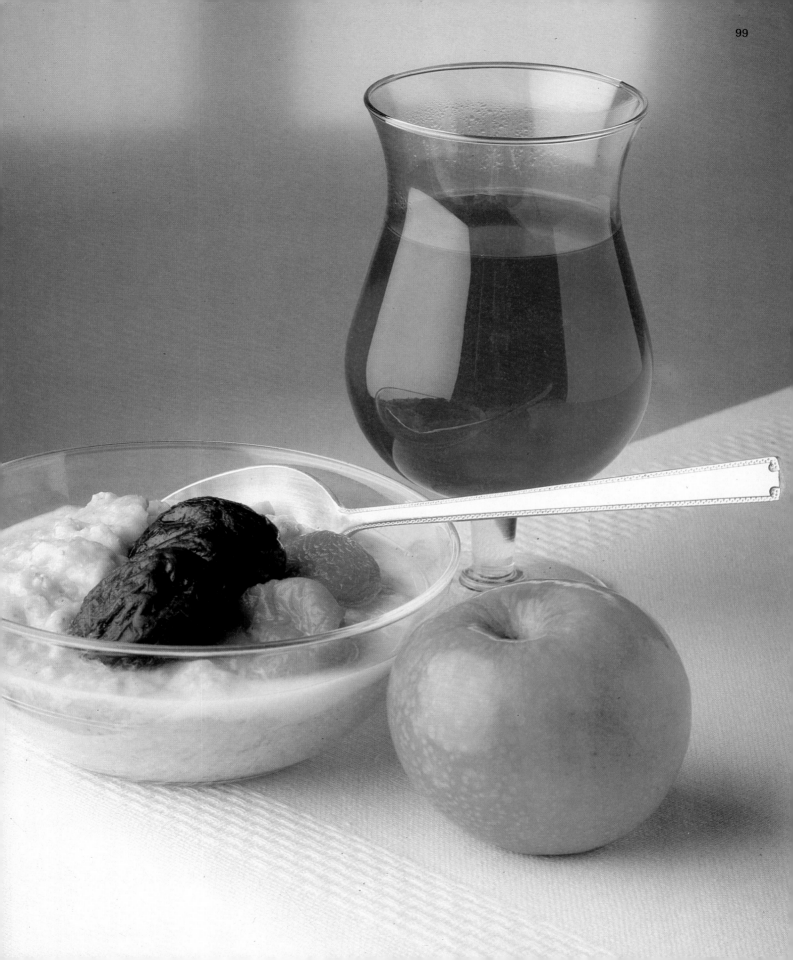

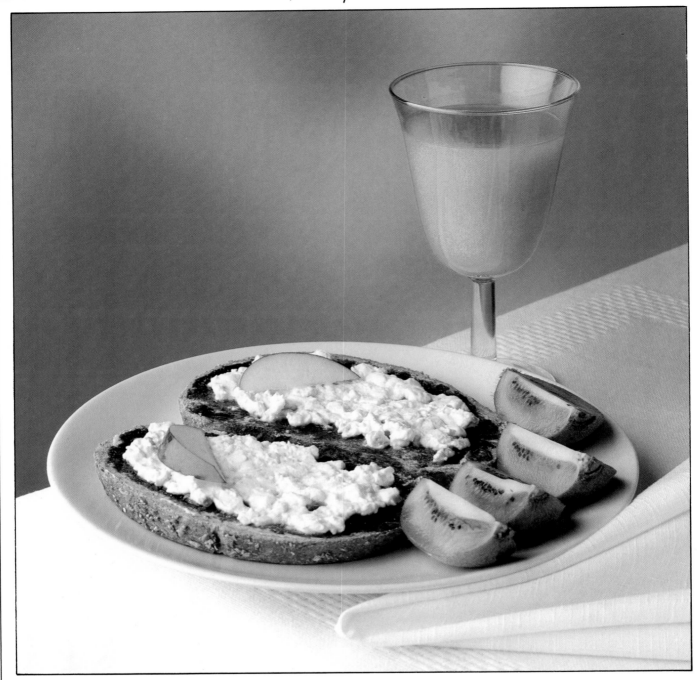

Above: breakfast 7: the bread isn't burnt, it's spread with yeast extract, a perfect flavour to go with cottage cheese. Swap the apricot nectar for your favourite juice, if liked, and sip slowly, you can add tea, herb or regular, without sweetening, if you like, or decaffeinated coffee.

1 *Total Calories 340*	*Approx. Cals.*	*Main food value*
2 good slices (2½oz total) wholemeal bread	155	protein, fibre, B vitamins, E, minerals
spread from allowance	–	fats, vitamins A and D
yeast extract topped with 2oz cottage cheese	70	protein, calcium, B vitamins, salt
1 large piece fruit or small banana	65	vitamin C, minerals (banana: vitamin A rather than C), fibre
small glass apricot nectar	50	vitamin A, minerals, fibre
drink from allowance if wanted	–	

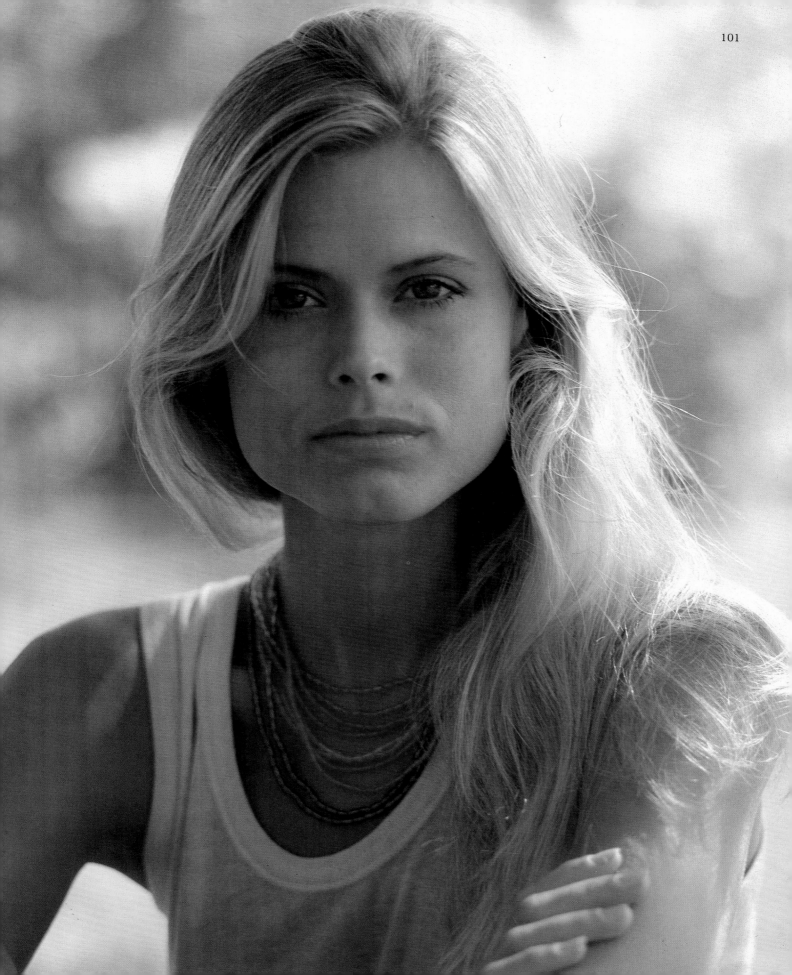

Light meals

Can be eaten midday or evening, as convenient. The exact quantities of vegetables are not given as calorie values are low enough to let you eat according to appetite without making much difference.

2 Burger platter:
calories around 410 including 90 for wine

Double decker Vegeburger on 2oz sesame wholemeal bun, sliced tomato, cucumber, spring onion
5oz glass of dry white wine

Vegetable burger mixes take only a few minutes to prepare to packet instructions. Grill or sauté in pan lightly brushed with oil.

4 Maxi-sandwich:
calories around 400

3 slices wholemeal bread
spread from allowance
filled with:
shredded carrot
yeast extract
3oz cottage cheese
sliced cucumber
side salad:
cauliflower chunks
carrot sticks
3oz unsweetened orange juice

Make bread into 3 super-filled sandwiches, using generous amounts of carrot and cucumber (plus watercress or mustard and cress if wanted).

Below: the maxi-sandwich that's mini in calories. Opposite: the burger platter – including a glass of wine. It's worth arranging meals prettily, even if they're just for you. You'll find you eat with more enjoyment and tend to feel satisfied with less.

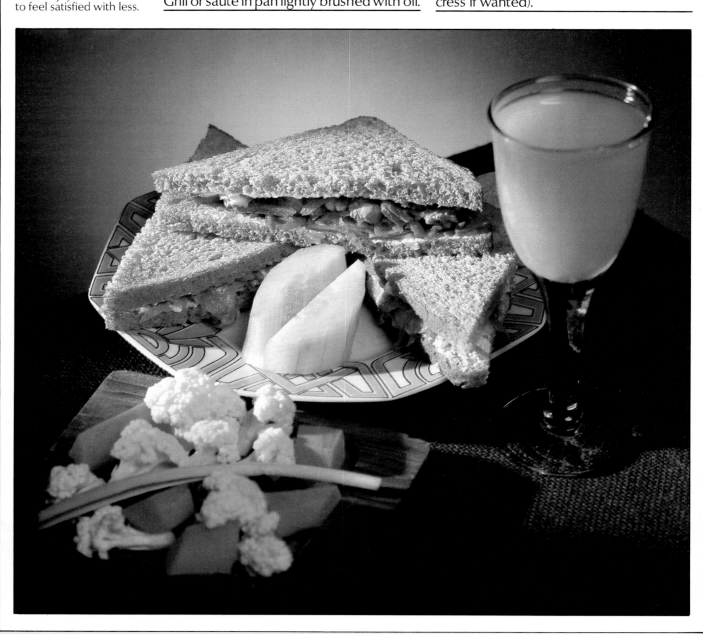

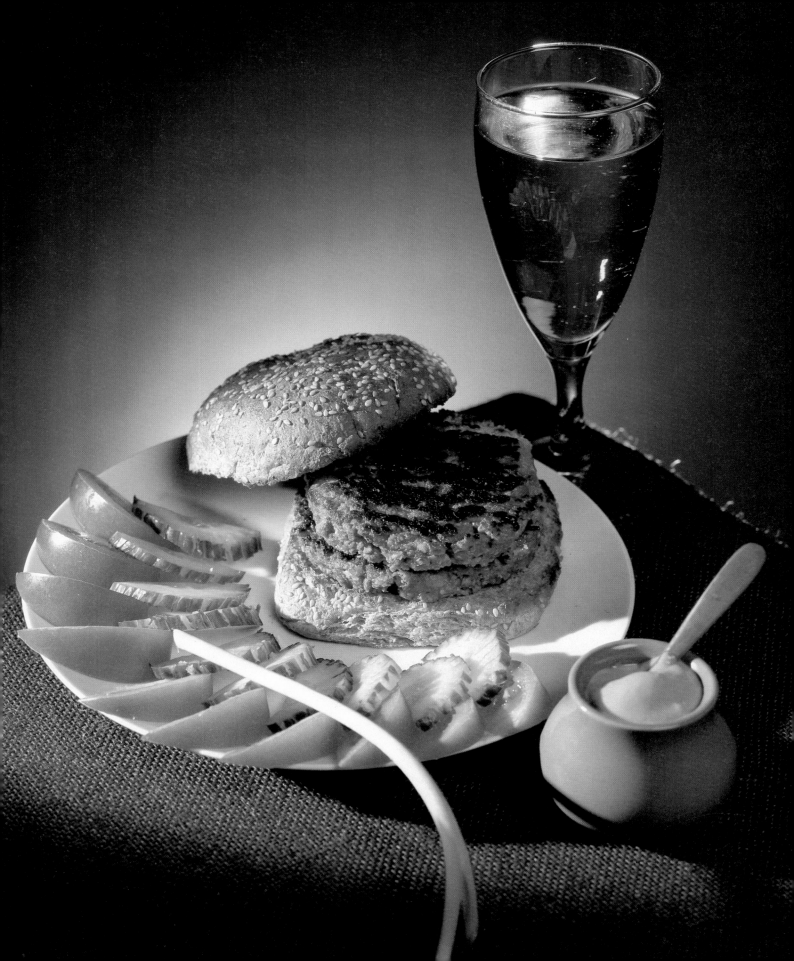

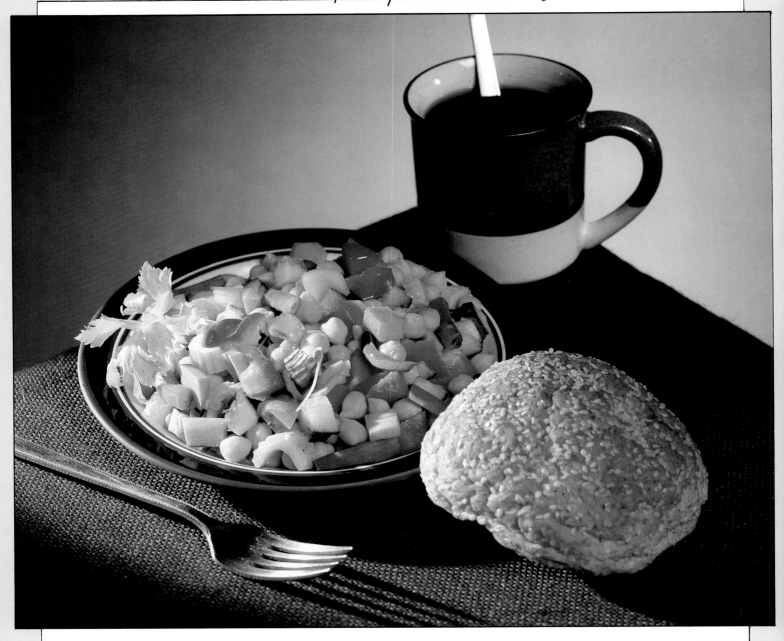

Above: the bean salad platter, good and crunchy with satisfying chick peas. Easy to take to work as these vegetables don't go soggy quickly. You can drink as many mugs of bouillon or yeast extract as you like: the calorie count is very low.
Opposite: the rice salad platter, much more filling made with brown rice. You can add more vegetables if you like. In cold weather, tomato juice is delicious hot.

1 Bean salad platter:
calories around 390

2oz chick peas or any dried bean
chopped fresh vegetables
2 tsp safflower or sunflower oil
good squeeze of lemon juice
2 tsp cider vinegar
1½oz wholemeal roll
Yeast extract hot drink

Soak beans in water overnight or during day. Change water, boil and simmer covered for about 40-60 minutes until tender. (Boil beans vigorously for 10 minutes before simmering.) Mix with all other ingredients while warm.

7 Rice salad platter:
calories around 340

2oz (raw weight) brown rice, cooked
½oz peanuts, toasted but not salted
½ bunch watercress, mustard and cress
or parsley
1 tbsp yogurt
squeeze of lemon juice
strips of green or red pepper
tomato juice with celery stick garnish

Cook rice as under Autumn salad. Mix with other ingredients, using vegetables generously.
Use yogurt as dressing.

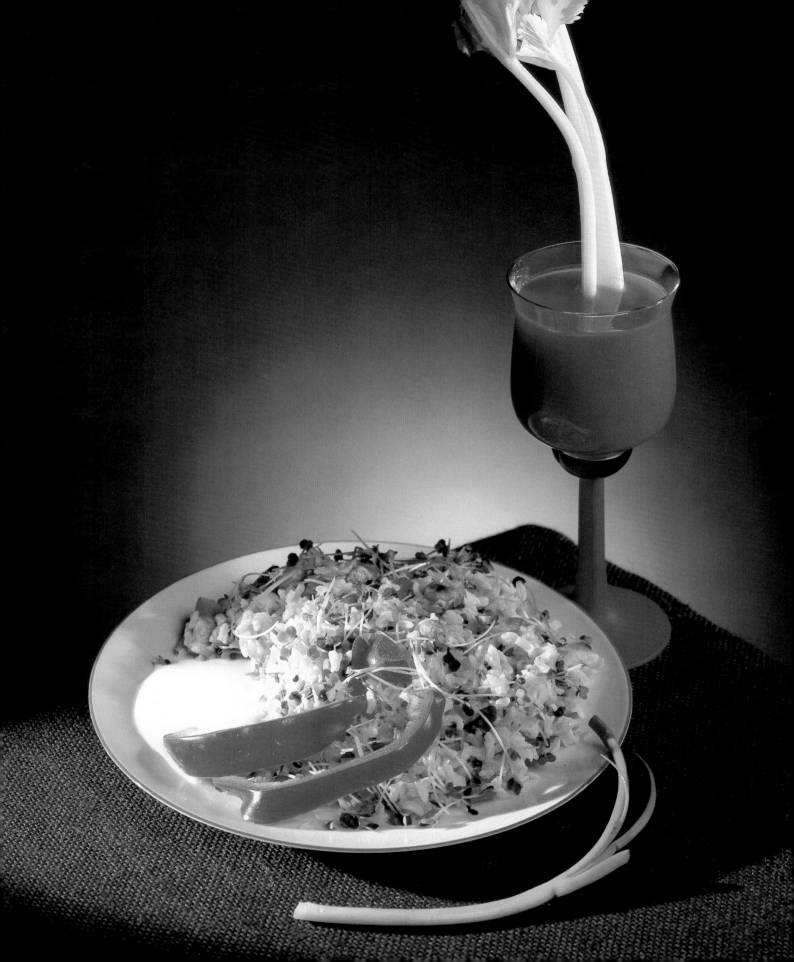

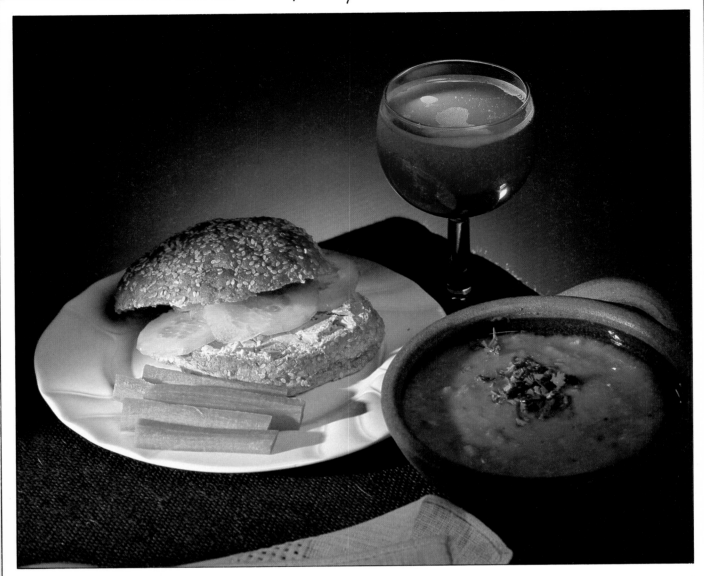

Above: Lentil soup with pate bap. Lentil soup is high in protein and fibre, as well as B vitamins, minerals and flavour! It can be kept hot in a vacuum flask without losing any goodness or taste. Opposite: baked potato platter allows you to enjoy a really big potato. You can keep it hot in a wide-mouthed vacuum flask, if wished, then add cottage cheese when you are ready to eat it.

5 Soup and pâté bap:
calories around 430

Lentil soup:
1 tsp vegetable oil
1 onion, finely sliced
1 carrot, washed and sliced
1oz split red lentils
1 bay leaf
¼ pint stock
sea salt and pepper to taste
yeast extract to taste

2oz wholemeal roll filled with ½oz Tartex[tm]
vegetable pâté
sliced cucumber
apple juice drink from concentrate

Heat oil in saucepan, soften onion with lid on for 5 minutes over lowest heat. Add carrot, lentils, bay leaf and stock. Simmer, covered, for 20 minutes.

Season, adding yeast extract if liked and more water if too thick. Remove bay leaf, liquidise. Transfer to vacuum flask if eating away from home.

6 Baked potato platter:
calories around 460

10oz baked potato
Coleslaw:
shred carrots, cabbage, add ½oz raisins
¼oz hazel nuts or sunflower seeds
3oz cottage cheese
½ bunch watercress or mustard and cress
Mineral water

Split potato, stuff with half the cottage cheeses (no butter!). Use rest of cheese to dress salad, with a squeeze of lemon juice if liked. Mix all salad ingredients together.

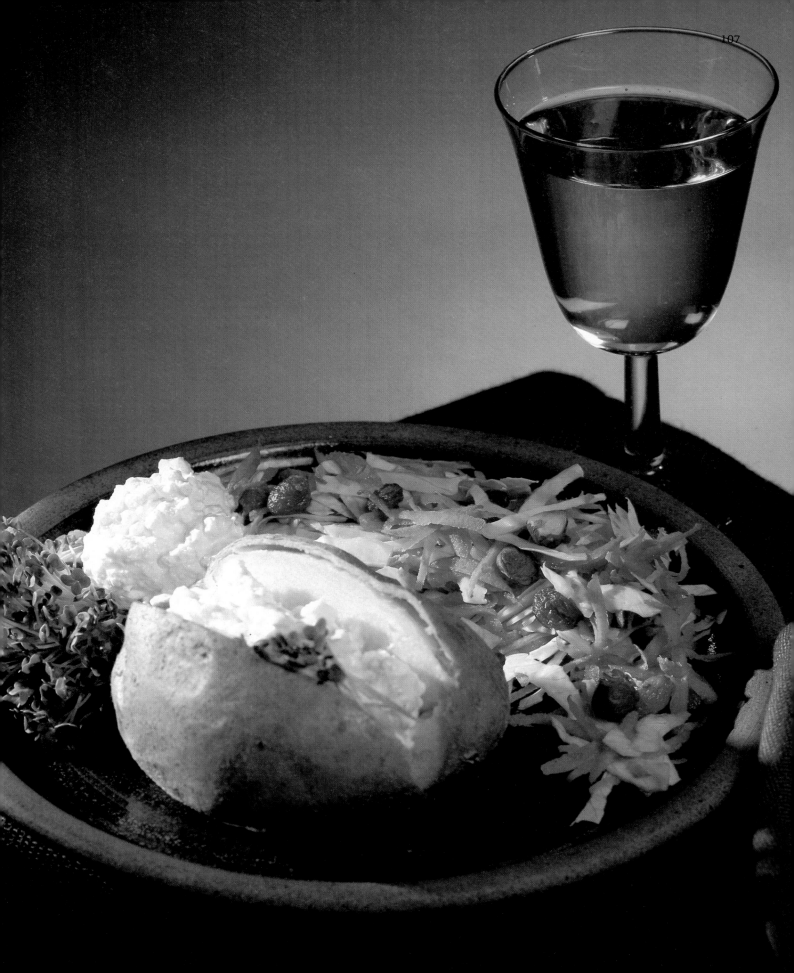

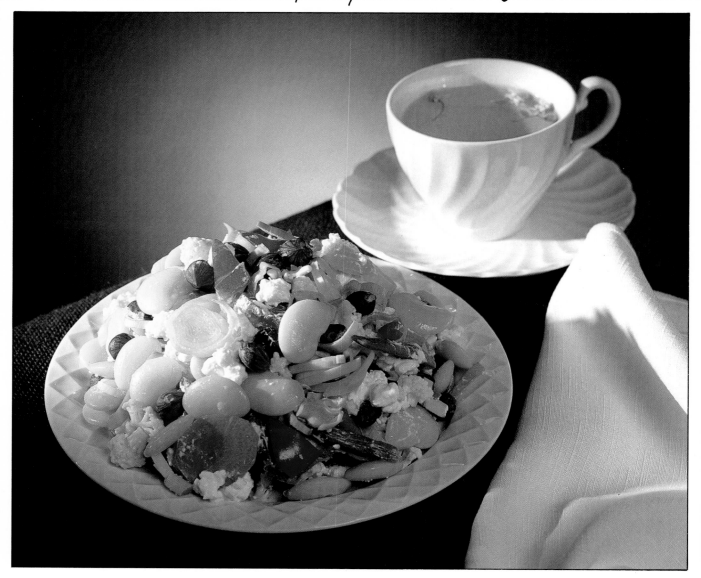

Above: autumn salad – a really generous plateful, with a delicate and relaxing cup of chamomile tea. Don't dismiss beans as too much trouble: cook a triple batch when you have time, then refrigerate or freeze until you want them for soups, casseroles or salad.

Opposite: younger women don't have all the cards. Mature good looks often go with greater self-confidence, serenity and the ability to enjoy life.

Autumn salad:
calories around 410

2oz (dry weight) beans or brown rice, cooked
generous selection of shredded vegetables, such as carrot, celery, leeks, cauliflower etc.
½oz hazel nuts, toasted but not salted
3oz cottage cheese or 1oz cheddar cheese
lemon juice or vinegar to flavour if liked
chamomile tea (or favourite herb tea)

Cook beans as for Bean salad; rice by simmering with 2½ times its volume of water, covered, for 40-50 minutes, when water will have been absorbed.
Mix with other ingredients, shredding cheddar cheese if used.

N.B. Hazel nuts have about 108 calories per ounce, compared to 150-170 for other nuts; this is due to their lower oil content.

Main Meals

Choose one of these:
* Medium portion of white fish, occasion-ally herring or kipper, and shellfish.
* Joint of chicken, turkey or rabbit; liver or kidneys at least once a week.
* Repeat any 'light meal'.
* Vegetables with skim milk white sauce and a little grated cheese.

Cook by baking, grilling or casseroling, i.e. don't add fat.
Add:
* 2 generous helpings of lightly cooked vegetables, 1 green (no potatoes)
* dessert of fresh fruit, or baked apple stuffed with dried fruit, or grilled grapefruit (pint type for preference) brushed with honey, or unsweetened yogurt with chopped fresh fruit.

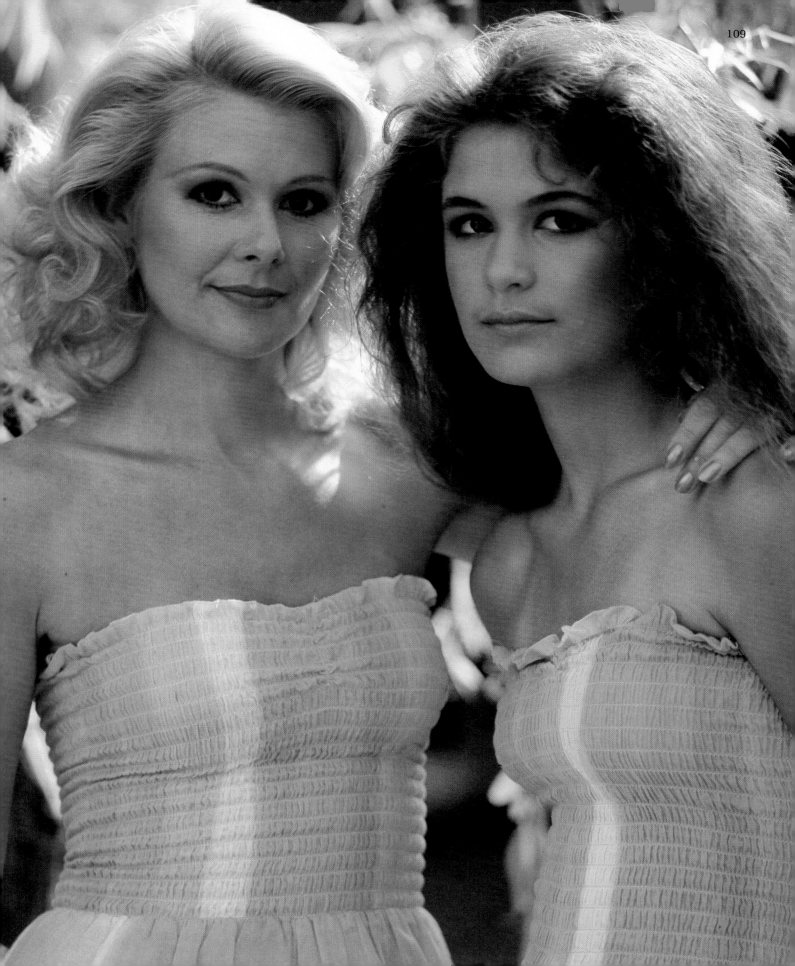

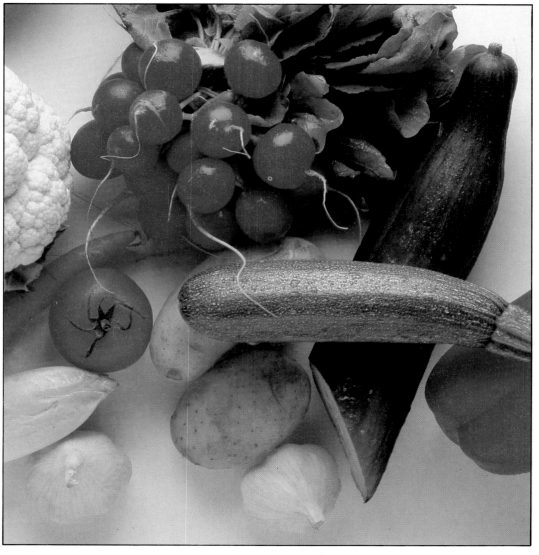

Above: an old trick, but it works. Keep a good stock of prepared (washed or peeled) vegetables chilled and handy for hungry moments when you might be tempted to dive into biscuits or ice cream. Opposite: a wide choice of drinks for flavour without calories or nerve-twitching caffeine. From top: chamomile tea – traditionally relaxing; top right: refreshing rosehip tea; next row, left: dandelion coffee, and opera singer's special (1 teaspoon each of honey, lemon juice and cider vinegar, with very hot water); bottom row, left: decaffeinated black coffee, lime flavoured tea, bouillon made with yeast extract.

✱ Drink from allowance.
Calories will average around 400.

'Free' Drinks
Too much caffeine and tannin from coffee, tea, cola drinks or chocolate can over-stimulate you and make you nervy. Therefore, try to use the following instead:
  Decaffeinated coffee
  Weak tea
  Dandelion and grain 'coffee'
  Lemon juice with hot water and 1 tsp honey, plus a dash of cider vinegar
  Tomato juice
  Lemon barley water (pour boiling water over lemon rind and barley in a jug, strain when cold, add minimum of honey to taste)
  Fruit juices, unsweetened – up to ½ pint a day.
  Fruit nectars, which are slightly sweetened, in small amounts.

  Mineral water.
  Vegetable cocktail juices.
  Herb teas, e.g. rosehip, chamomile, peppermint, fennel, mixed fruit.
  Apple juice, including drinks made from juice concentrate with hot or cold water.
  Glass of dry wine not more than 3 times a week. Try making it go further by mixing with sparkling mineral water.

'Free' Vegetables
All vegetables provide good food value per calorie, but to control weight use freely all but the following: sweet corn, sweet potatoes, peas, baked beans, broad beans. Use small amounts of these, but avoid avocado pears completely if calorie-counting; they are very high indeed, thanks to their oil content.

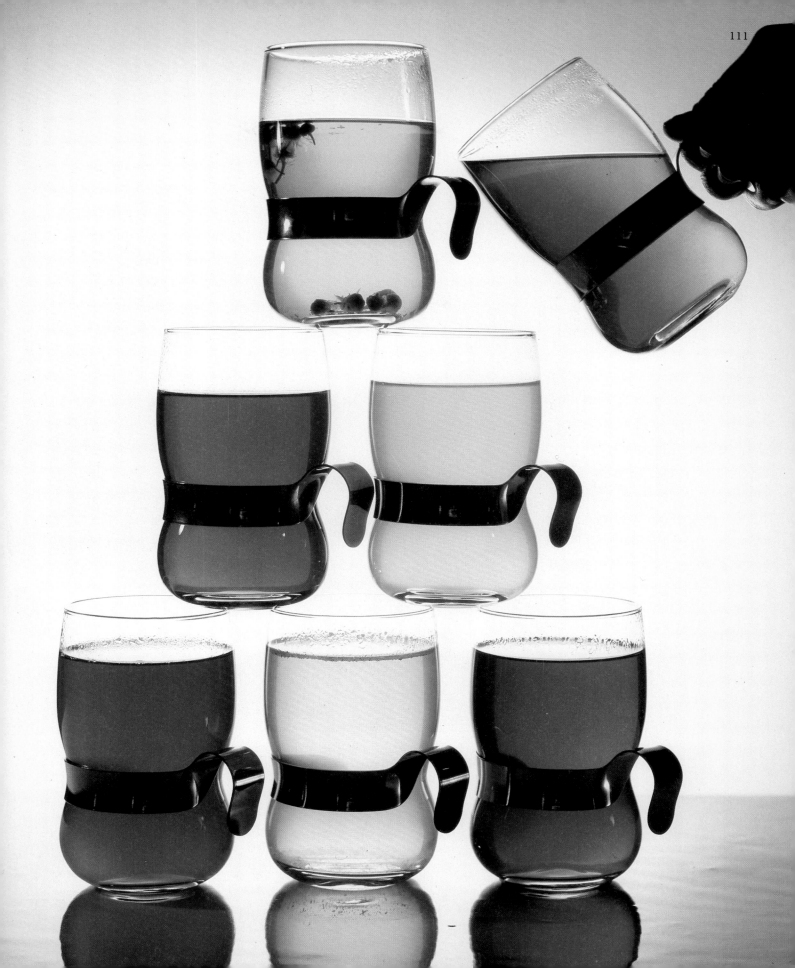

CHAPTER 9

Eating well away from Home

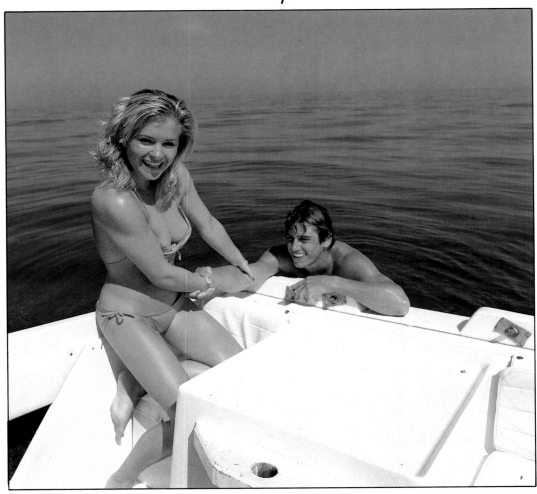

Right and opposite: many of us make an effort to eat healthily and get in shape at home, then give up when we go away. But the food that makes us feel confident in our swimwear can taste just as delicious as the stuff that brings out the spots and bulges.

Business lunches, holidays and having to eat out are all used as reasons for not being able to eat healthily. It's true that they do present you with many dishes which are richer in fat, sugar and salt than you might eat at home, but you'd be surprised how many healthy foods are there for the choosing.

Holidays: apply the same yardsticks as at home. You want to avoid excess fat and sugar, but increase fibre, fruit and vegetables. So choose salads (easy when it's hot), fish, poultry and fruit rather than fried or sugary dishes. That could mean, for instance, picking a *tjatziki* (cucumber and yogurt) dish if you're in Greece, rather than the high fat *tyropitta* pastries as your first course, and going for the many bean and vegetable dishes on offer, rather than fried food. Fish is good at most seaside holiday places, but opt for it grilled, barbecued or casseroled rather than fried in batter; or leave the batter aside.

Avoiding meat and rich puddings will also reduce your chances of getting food

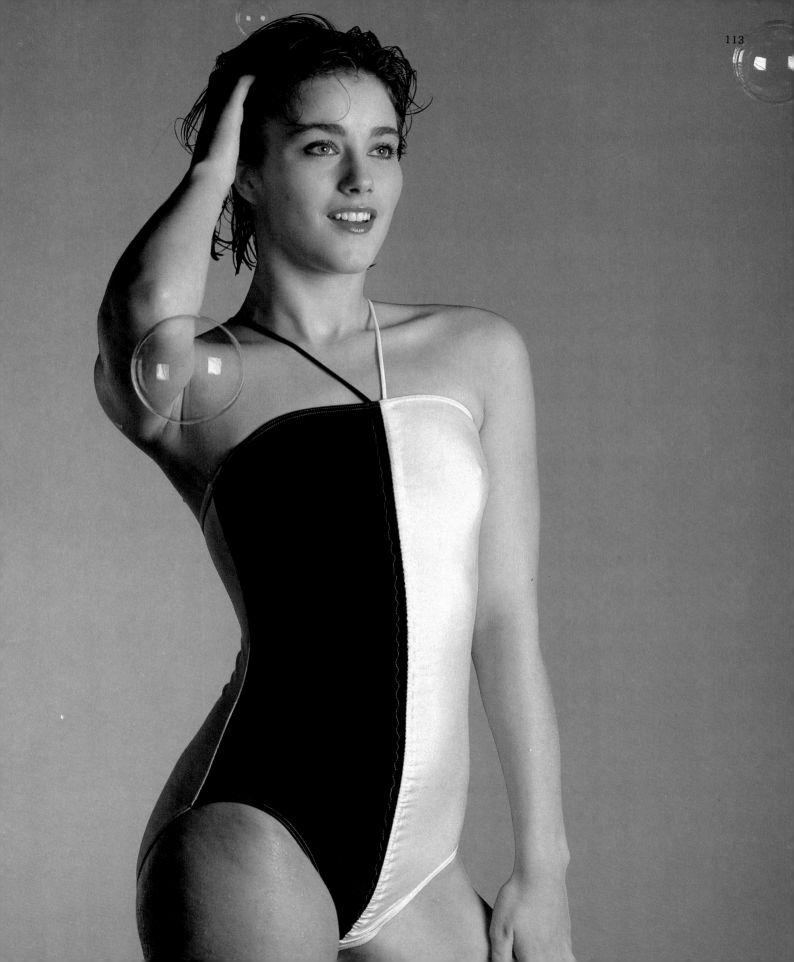

Below: dessert trolley temptation! There's always fresh fruit salad or fresh pineapple, or a simple 'no', which may be hard to say but you'll soon be pleased you did.
A moment in the mouth, an hour in the stomach, a lifetime on the hips...
If you seldom eat puddings,

poisoning, which is more liable to affect animal foods like cream, custard, ice cream and meat.

Look out for local specialities such as corn on the cob (avoid the butter or most of it), melons, or barbecued food, which reduces fat. You'll often find it hard to find wholemeal bread or cereal, so it can be worth taking with you packets of pumpernickel,

Business lunches: it's never been so easy to avoid the business paunch! Restaurants are increasingly catering for the health-minded. However, you may have to make a few requests; don't be nervous, they'll accept it as normal. Ask for salad dressings to be served separately, so you can control the amount you add. Ask for sauces to be left off dishes like seafood cocktail or

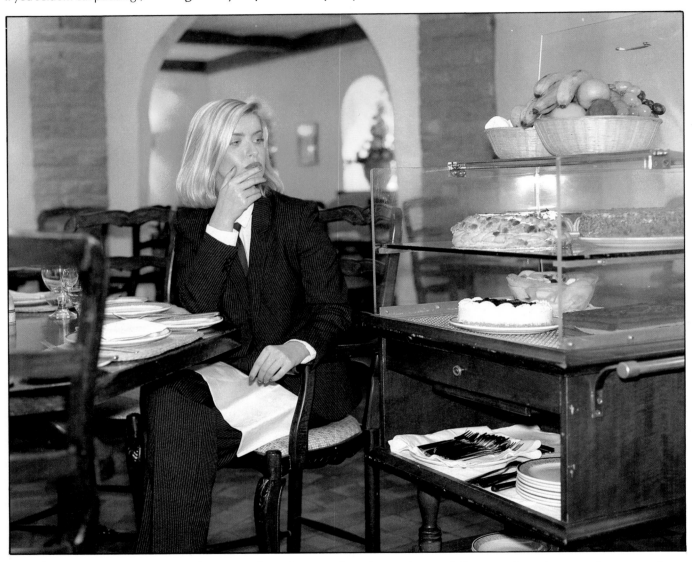

or confectionery say once a month, then of course you can say 'yes' cheerfully. But once you are used to healthy eating, you may not want to.

Opposite: the grandest food, like caviar, smoked salmon or fresh raspberries, can be healthy, too.

which keeps well until opened, and muesli (sugar-free brand). If you are going self-catering, you can take you own brown rice and pasta, for instance.

To stay well on holiday, don't eat fruit unless you've peeled it yourself. Don't drink unboiled water or have ice in drinks, and be wary of seafood around the polluted Mediterranean. Alcohol and sun are a potent mixture which can lead to tummy upsets all on their own, especially if you drink an unfamiliar local brew.

puddings, and again served separately so you can reduce the amount you eat. Ask for sauces on main courses, like fish, to be reduced or omitted; they usually consist of butter and cream.

Easy-to-find first courses include: melon, grapefruit cocktail, seafood cocktail without dressing, thin soups, mixed salads, oysters, asparagus (with only a drop of dressing), artichoke (ditto), moules marinière (mussels), crudites (raw vegetable sticks with a dip – ask for cottage

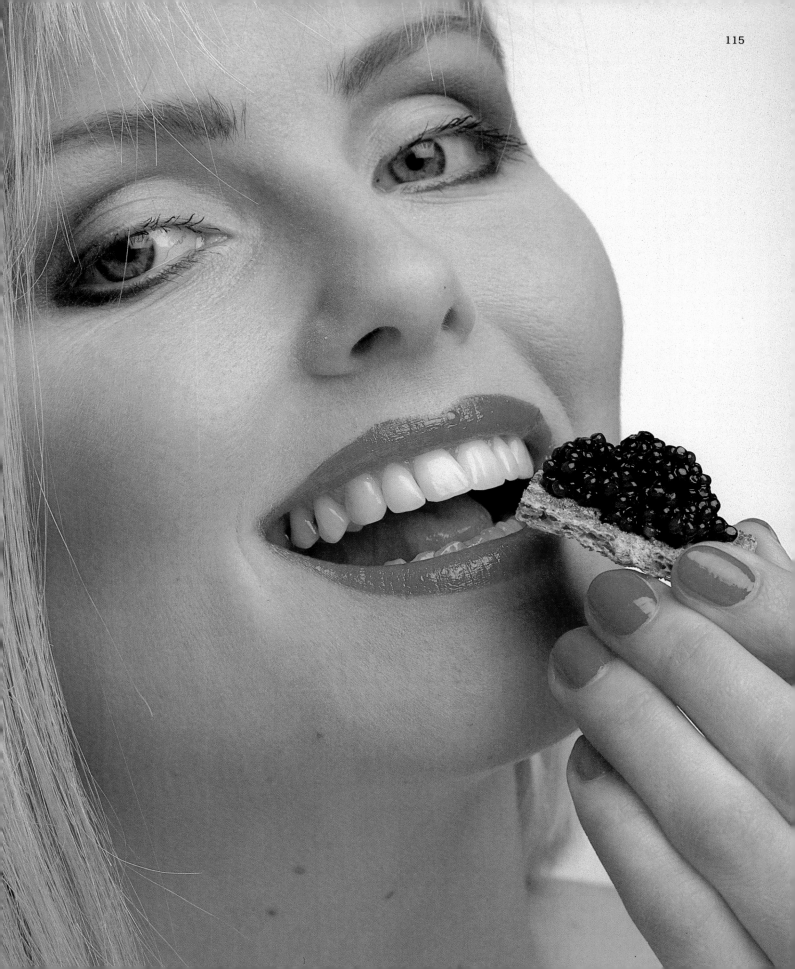

cheese instead, or use dip cautiously), and smoked fish.

Main courses: pick a plain poultry, fish, game or rabbit dish, with vegetables (ask for them not to be buttered). More restaurants now offer vegetarian main dishes, but avoid fried croquettes, rich in nut oil. Choose jacket-baked or boiled potatoes, rather than creamed or chipped, and in preference to white rice or white noodles.

Puddings: try eating fresh fruit salad, fresh fruit such as raspberries, strawberries, orange sliced in liqueur or stewed figs, crème caramelle or crumble, leaving most of the topping. Don't pick cheese and biscuits unless you've had a very light meal, such as a salad.

persuade you, resist; why should you drink more than you want? Alcohol provides 'empty calories' and can't help your health or your looks.

Take-Aways Most of us want a take-away meal at some time. Here's the choice you'll usually have; which is best for your health?

Baked potato (9oz) with baked beans (2½oz). If you ask for the pat of butter to be omitted, totals about 265 calories. Excellent for health with vitamin C from potato, plus fibre, minerals and protein with B vitamins, fibre and minerals for beans.
Fried chicken pieces (9½oz) with chips (4½oz). Poor health choice, with too much fat and little fibre. A little vitamin C is found in the chips. Contains around 800 calories.
Double cheeseburger (4oz meat) with

The take-away choice. Top row from left: baked potato with baked beans; fried chicken with chips; cheeseburger and milk-shake; pork pie and stout; coffee and Danish pastries. Bottom row from left: frankfurter with fried onions; chicken chop suey, pizza, doner kebab; vegetable curry with chapattis; tuna and cucumber sandwich; fish and chips.

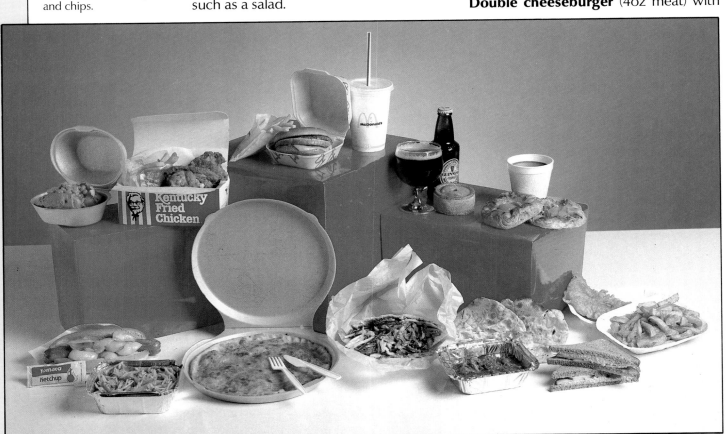

Opposite: how can you expect to look as alive as this if you eat too much fatty, sugary, packaged food?

Coffee: ask for decaffeinated. More restaurants now offer it and, if more of us ask for it, they all will. Otherwise, carry sachets of decaffeinated coffee or herb tea in your pocket, and ask them to make them up. You can always plead your doctor's advice!
Alcohol: stick to a glass or two of dry wine, remembering that more will blunt your business judgement (it is a working lunch, isn't it?) as well as your health. If they try to

1oz cheese, chips (2¼oz) and 2oz bun. Thin chips like these tend to be highest in fat in proportion to amount of potato. No vitamin C in this one, almost no fibre, with plenty of fat. Contains around 880 calories, including milk shake. Only advantage: plenty of protein, from hamburger, cheese, bun and shake's milk content.
Bottle of stout (275ml) and pork pie (5oz). One of the worst choices, providing some 628 calories, of which a high

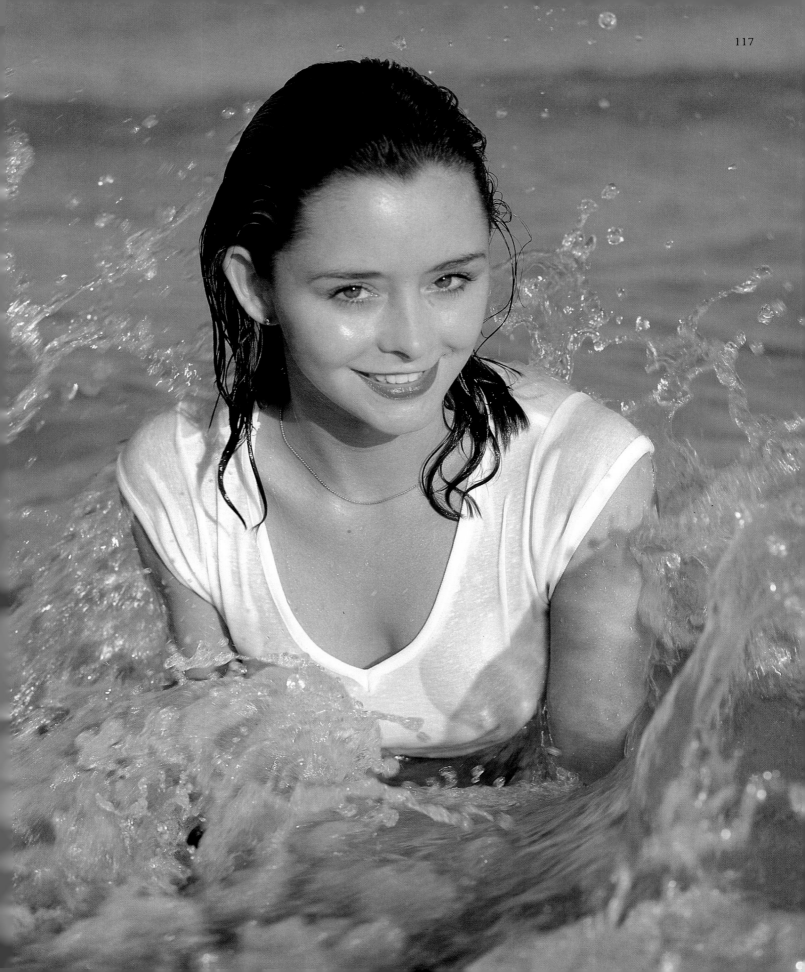

proportion come from fat. Virtually no fibre, no vitamin C at all, few vitamins and minerals compared to what the same number of calories would provide in the form of other foods.

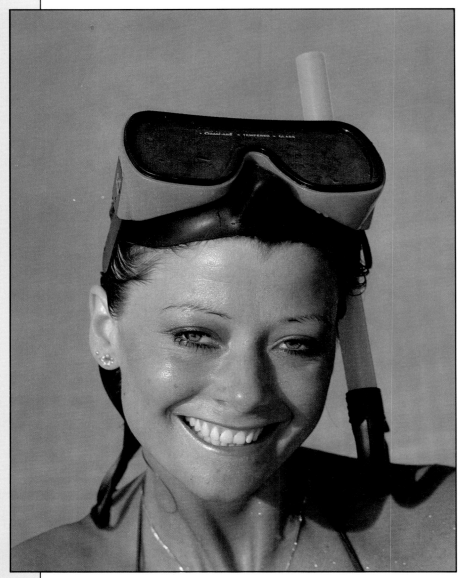

Keep a note of what to look for in food value – low fat, freshness, wholemeal or bean-based dishes for fibre, and you'll be able to choose the healthiest of what's available wherever you travel. Remember basic rules too: avoid unboiled water, including ice in drinks, peel fruit and vegetables, refuse seafood unless you're very confident.

Cup of coffee and Danish pastries. With 14ml cream from the standard portion tub and 6oz for the pastries, this provides a colossal 1,000-odd calories, is mainly fat and has almost no fibre and no vitamin C. Bottom of the list, and the coffee may also make you feel nervy!

Hot dog. A 4oz frankfurter in a typical 2¾oz roll with 1½oz fried onion provides roughly 625 calories, complete with protein but little else apart from fat. Virtually no fibre or vitamin C.

Pizza. An 8oz slice of pizza or complete pizza made with wholemeal flour (easier to find now) provides about 520 calories, with

around 11% fat. Cheese and flour provide the protein, and there's vitamin C in tomato topping (ask for peppers – they're very high in vitamin C), and the base also provides fibre. This is one of the best choices.

Chicken chop suey. This will vary from one restaurant to another but, basically, the Chinese stir-frying method results in a low fat result and chicken is one of the meats lowest in fat, especially as most restaurants remove the fattiest part, the skin. A 12oz portion might provide 4oz chicken, 8oz mixed vegetables – which should supply some vitamin C and fibre – and a typical 300 calories; a good choice.

Doner kebab, salad and pitta bread. With 3oz of each, this provides about 440 calories. The salad provides vitamin C and a little fibre and, if the pitta bread were wholemeal (now available), the meal would be well-balanced, because the fat content is low and the bread would then provide more fibre and vitamins.

Vegetable curry and 2 chapattis. A 9oz curry will vary considerably in food value according to the cook's use of fat and length of cooking time for the vegetables. It provides some fibre and a little vitamin C, for about 400 calories. Many Indian restaurants use wholemeal flour for chapattis, which would make this a good meal as it's relatively low in fat, if you supplied the vitamin C with an orange for afters.

Tuna and cucumber sandwich in wholemeal bread. With about 2½oz tuna and little butter or margarine, this clocks up about 330 calories, complete with protein, vitamin C from the cucumber and fibre from the bread. A very good choice, especially if you ask for extra salad to be included.

Fish and chips. A generous 7oz fish and 10oz chips gave this meal a solid 1,266 calories! This amount of chips would provide some fibre and a good helping of vitamin C, but an awful lot of fat with it. If you peeled the batter off the fish, you'd be peeling off a lot of the fat too. Keep this one for special occasions.

Summary of Best Buys:
✻ Baked potato with baked beans
✻ Tuna and cucumber wholemeal sandwich
✻ Chicken chop suey
✻ Vegetable curry with wholemeal chapattis

Runners-Up Pizza and doner kebab would be good if wholemeal, and pizza needs salad for vitamin C.

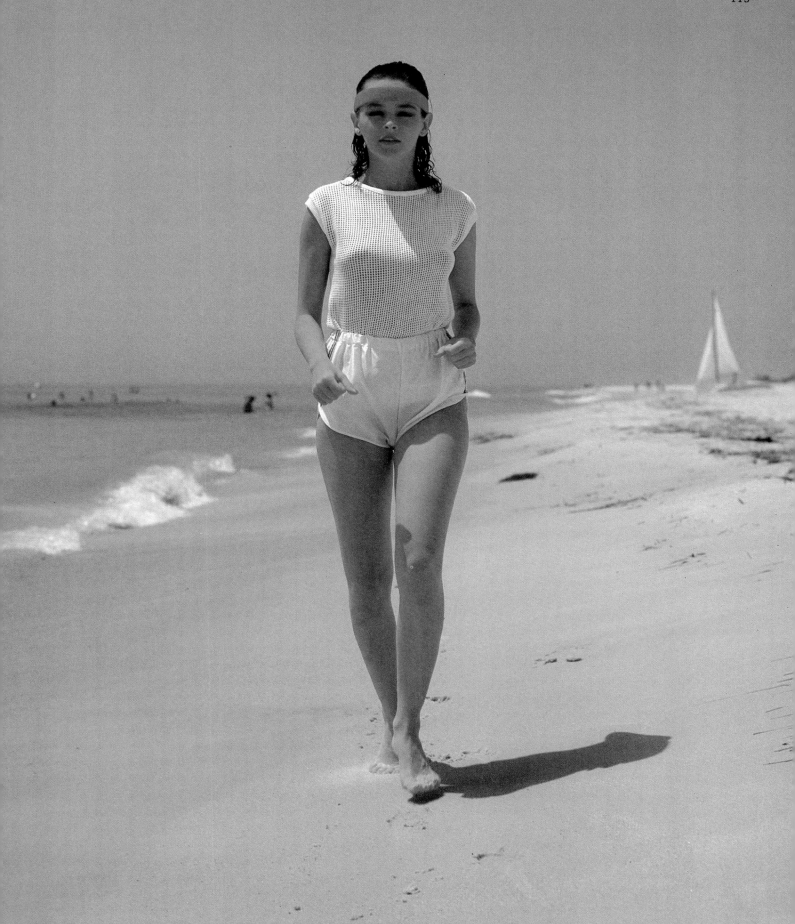

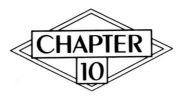

CHAPTER 10

Exercise and Relaxation

Opposite: your leg and stomach muscles can take the strain; if you keep your back straight, bend your legs. Learning how to keep your back happy is crucial to fitness.

Food can't be discussed without taking into account the other side of the balance: the energy we use.

Exercise has benefits you may not have considered. As well as helping to control your weight, and keeping you in shape with trim muscles, exercise can:

* Increase your energy level, by making your body stronger.

* Improve your stamina.

* Help you resist stress by improving stamina and helping you relax.

* Mean you can eat more while staying in shape. The more you eat, provided you choose natural foods, the more vitamins and minerals you'll be eating too, to supply your body with materials for good health. Lots of people also find another benefit worth having from exercise; it puts them in a good mood!

You don't have to be a natural athlete or fanatical sports fan to benefit.

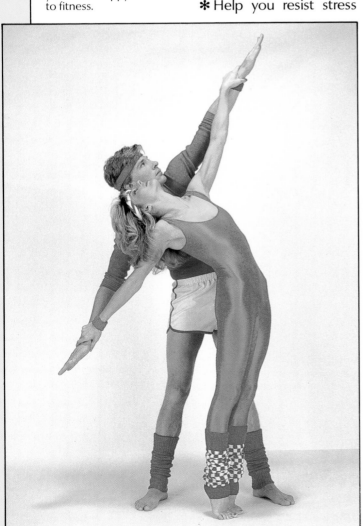

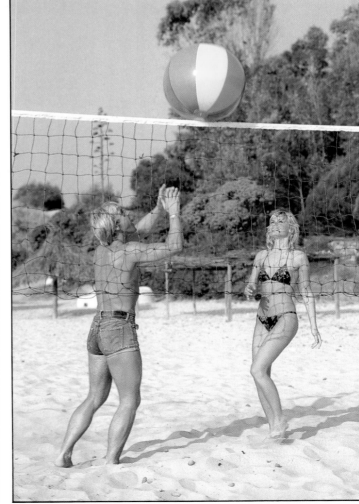

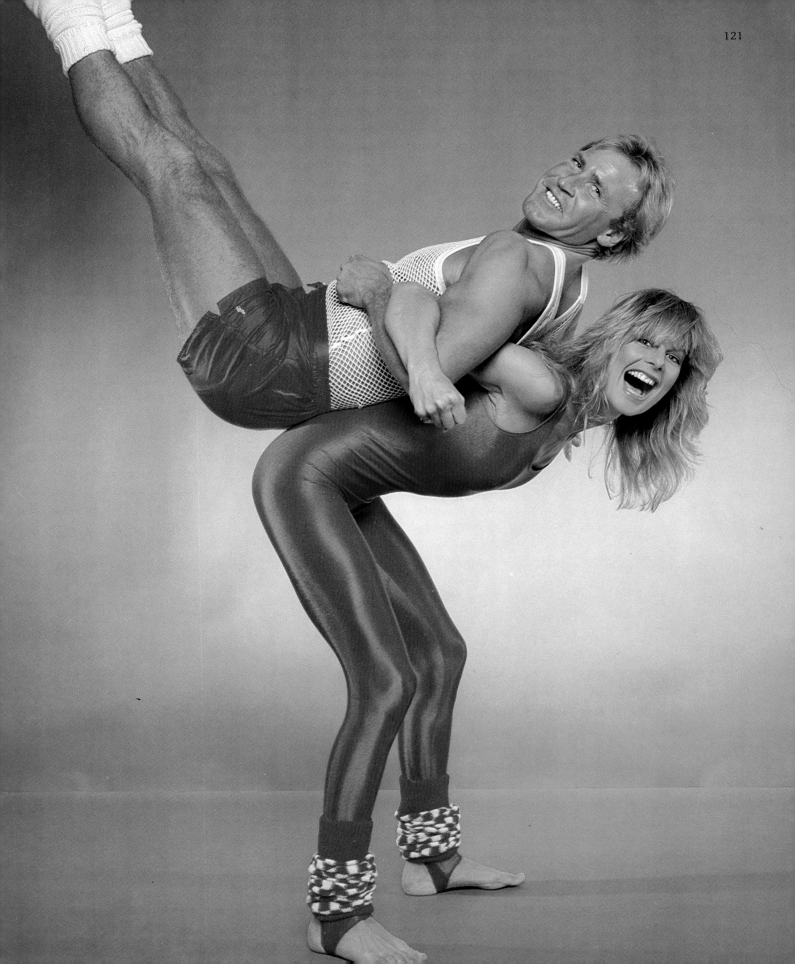

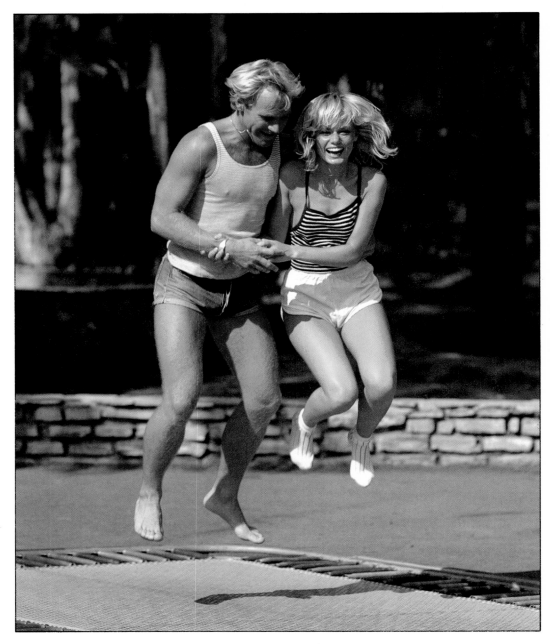

When people talk about aerobics, they simply mean exercise which increases the body's need for oxygen. A sure sign of that happening is getting hot – and that's a simple target to aim for when choosing how active to be!
To be safe from overstrain, don't be competitive; take breaks, treat it as fun, don't go on when you feel tired.

Exercise experts agree that the most valuable exercise for almost everyone, no matter what their age or fitness, is **swimming**, because it uses many muscles in a situation where you are unlikely to hurt yourself. Three sessions of 20-30 minutes a week can improve your stamina, especially if you swim with concentration and don't just splash around.

Next best comes **walking**, provided it is brisk. It has the advantage that you can do it anywhere and every day, so although it doesn't have such a high rating for energy use, the amount you do will build up to something useful. Include some hills or stairs for maximum benefit.

Cycling is another exercise which many people can fit into their daily routine, so increasing its beneficial effect on their fitness. Mainly benefits the lower half of your body and, as you don't want to be schizophrenic – with a fit bottom, but flabby top – ideally combine it with another kind of exercise.

Bouncing on a mini-trampoline is a bit like jogging on the spot, with less risk of foot and ankle jar or injury, because you land on a surface that 'gives'. Exercises your heart, lower half of your body and shakes out tension.

Dancing: this doesn't have to be dazzling stuff to keep you fit. Ballroom, disco, folk or

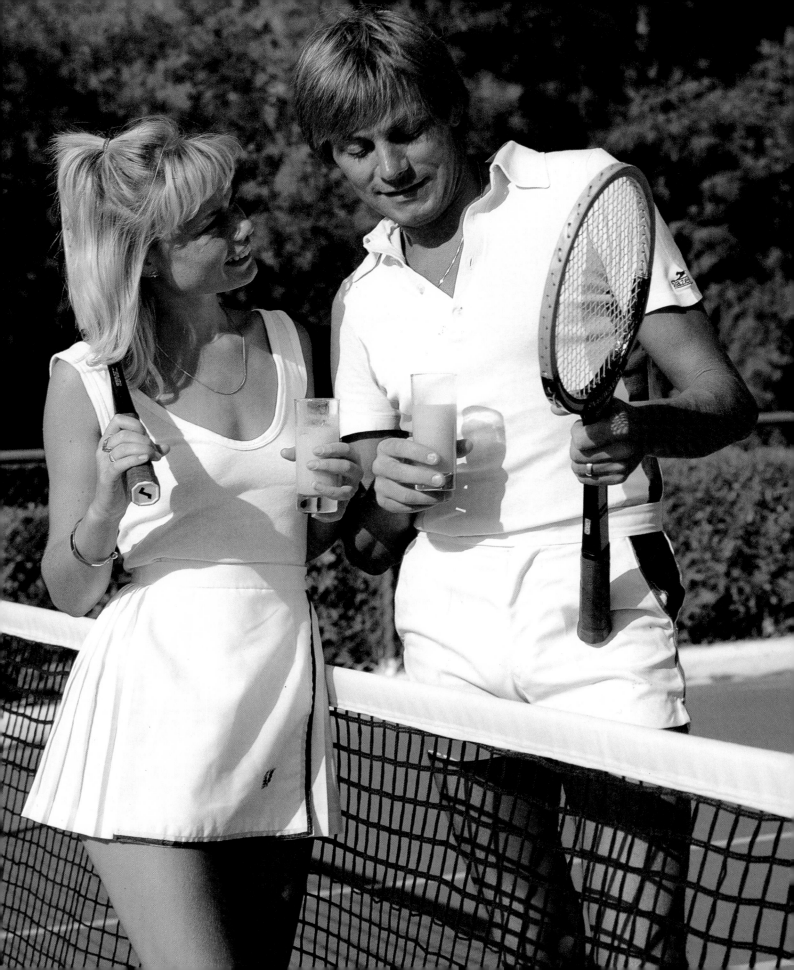

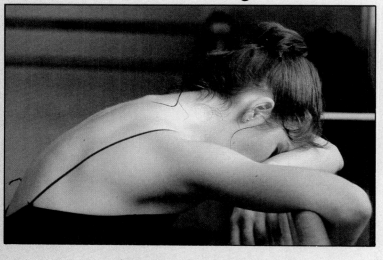

Relaxation

How relaxed you are will affect both your attitude to food and the use your body can make of it. Anxious people don't digest as well and are more inclined to eat poorly, or to binge on sweet foods; both of which should be avoided.

Exercise of all kinds can help you relax, both by shaking the tension out of your muscles as you move and by giving your mind a rest. It must be exercise, though,

ballet dancing will all tone up muscles and heart capacity if done to the extent where you get hot and breathless.

Housework: varies in its exercise value. Scrubbing the floor and polishing are excellent; dusting is not so hot. Just going up and down stairs is good exercise. Put your back into the household chores: stretch, bend, rub hard, and you'll be toning muscles without realising it.

Exercise classes: certainly tone muscles and help use up calories. However, choose them carefully, avoiding anything that's intended for people fitter than you. Injuries are common and can plague you for a long time. The most important element of a class is proper attention to warming up muscles, so you don't jerk or tear them when you exercise.

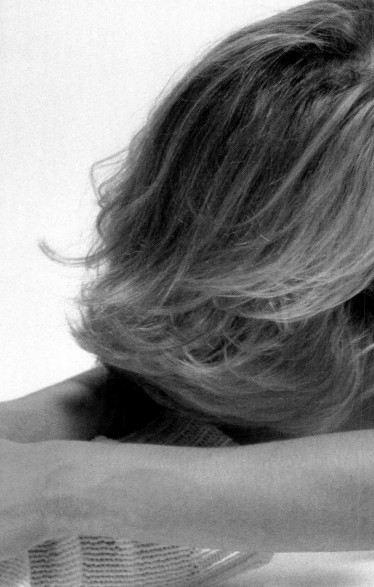

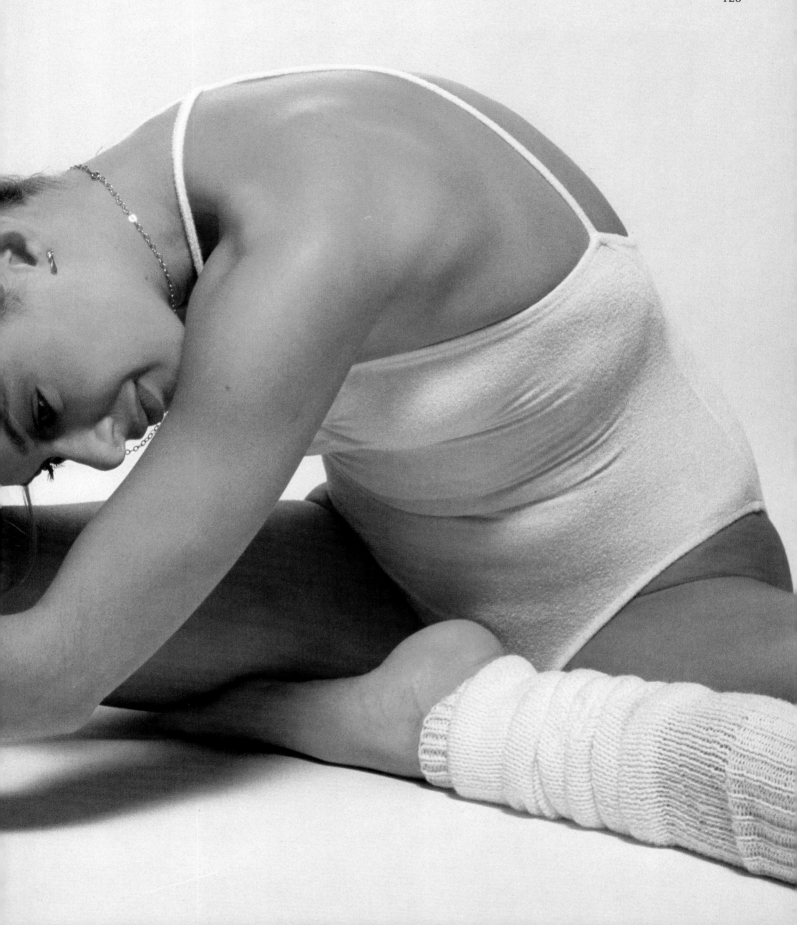

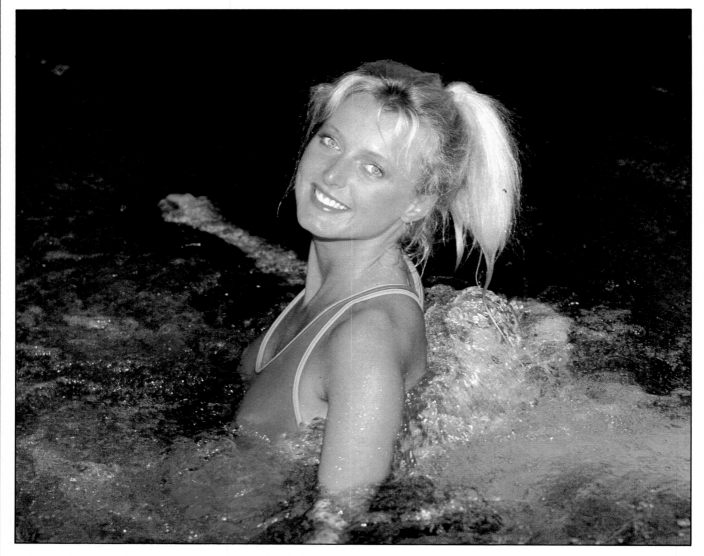

Swimming is accepted as the ideal form of exercise. Jacuzzi baths don't provide exercise – although they are ideal places in which to perform stretching exercises, as your muscles will be very relaxed. Relaxation is the main attraction, as with massage, and its health value should not be underestimated when so many health problems, from mental tension to backache, are related to stress.

that keeps your mind fully occupied, so you can't carry on worrying at the same time.

Have You Considered?

* **Breathing lessons**: shallow breathing encourages anxiety and rations the body's oxygen supply. Deep breathing is essential to relaxation and can be learned from classes or tapes.

* **Yoga**: is one of the most widely-available relaxation techniques, particularly useful for breathing and for learning how to put problems in perspective. By increasing your body awareness, it can also encourage you to eat more healthily.

* **Massage**: can help you relax. If you live with someone, why not both learn and treat each other?

* **Relaxation exercises**: can be learned at classes or from books. Again, they emphasize breathing, but can also point out to you personal habits that bring

tension, such as the way you sit or stand, which you may be unaware of but which can be changed for the better.

* **Water therapies**: from Turkish baths, saunas, jacuzzis and sitz baths to health farm-type underwater massage and herb baths, can help your muscles relax with warmth and rubbing. Sitz baths, which alternate hot and cold water showers or put one half of you in cold water, the other half in hot, then change round, improve circulation, as do saunas which also alternate hot and cold.

* **Hobbies**: like gardening are relaxing in three ways. They use up your attention, so you can't worry about daily life; they provide fresh air, and they give you something life-enhancing and beautiful to think about. Looking after animals outdoors, bird-watching, flower-photography and watercolour painting are among other pursuits with these benefits.

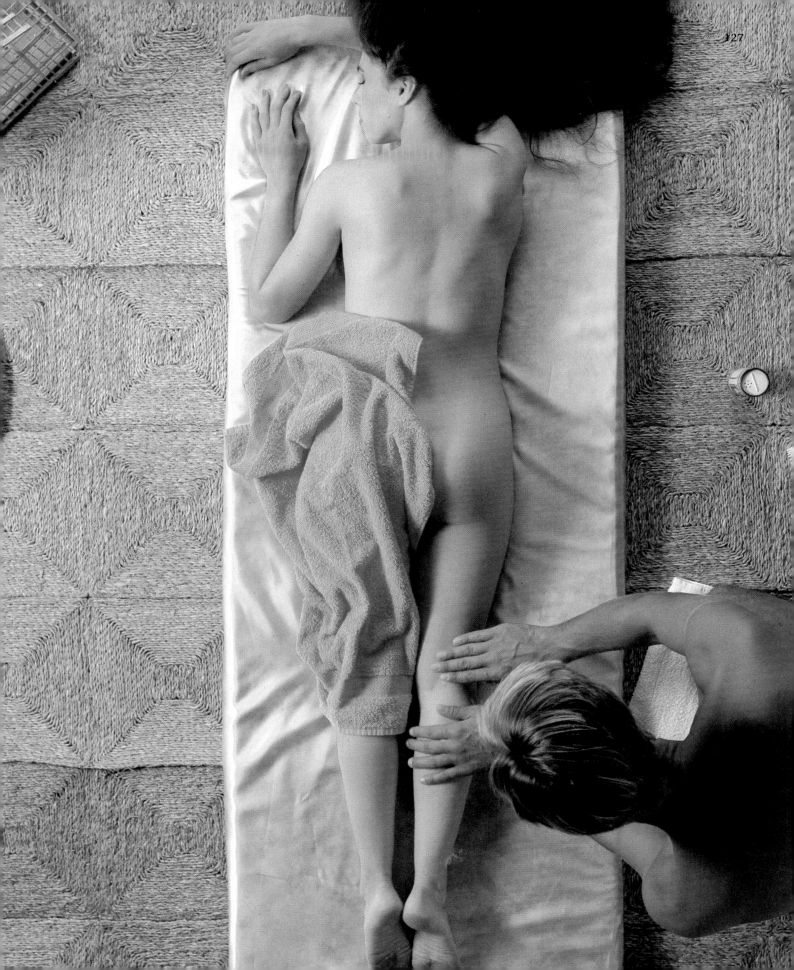

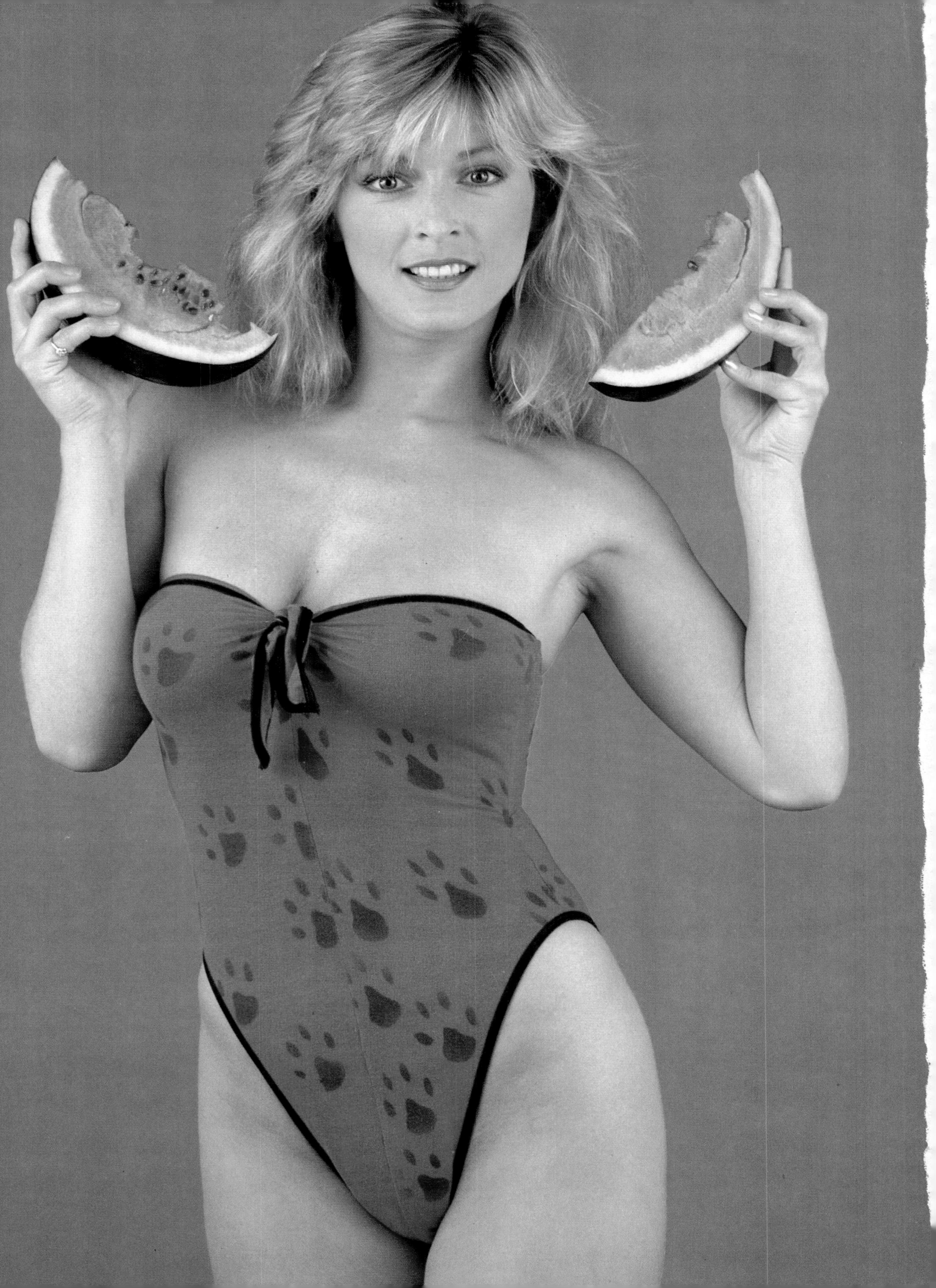